The Updated Parkinson's Diet Therapy 2024

By

Calvin M. Duncan

Table of Contents

Introduction

Parkinson's Disease (PD), a complex neurodegenerative disorder, not only challenges the motor functions of those affected but also necessitates a holistic approach to care. Amidst the multifaceted strategies employed for managing Parkinson's, the role of diet emerges as a pivotal component in promoting overall well-being, potentially influencing symptom progression, and enhancing the quality of life for individuals navigating this challenging journey.

The brain, the epicenter of Parkinson's pathology, requires a continuous supply of nutrients to function optimally. Nutritional choices play a crucial role in providing the brain with the building blocks it needs for maintaining cellular health and combating the impact of neurodegeneration.

A well-rounded diet that includes a balance of macronutrients—carbohydrates, proteins, and fats—is fundamental. Carbohydrates serve as the primary energy source, providing the fuel needed for daily activities. Whole grains, fruits, and vegetables not only supply energy but also contribute essential vitamins and minerals.

Proteins, comprising amino acids, are vital for the synthesis of neurotransmitters—chemical messengers crucial for communication between nerve cells. However, protein intake in Parkinson's requires thoughtful consideration, as some individuals may experience interactions between protein and medication absorption. Collaborative discussions with healthcare professionals help tailor protein consumption to individual needs.

Healthy fats, including omega-3 fatty acids found in fish, flaxseeds, and walnuts, contribute to brain health. These fats possess anti-inflammatory properties, potentially mitigating the neuroinflammation associated with Parkinson's.

Parkinson's is characterized, in part, by oxidative stress—a state where the balance between free radicals and antioxidants is disrupted, leading to cellular damage. Antioxidant-rich foods, such as berries, leafy greens, and nuts, serve as defenders against oxidative stress, potentially offering a protective shield for neurons.

Vitamins C and E, both potent antioxidants, are found in abundance in fruits and vegetables. Incorporating these nutrient-rich foods into the diet contributes not only to overall health but also to the potential modulation of oxidative processes within the brain.

Adequate hydration is often overlooked but is integral to overall health. Proper hydration supports cellular functions, aids in medication absorption, and helps prevent complications such as constipation—a common issue in Parkinson's. Individuals are encouraged to maintain a consistent fluid intake, considering factors such as medication schedules and the potential impact of certain medications on fluid balance.

The intricate interplay between diet and medication in Parkinson's underscores the importance of informed choices. Levodopa, a primary medication for managing motor symptoms, requires careful consideration in terms of timing and dietary interactions. Protein consumption, for example, may affect the absorption of levodopa, prompting strategic planning of meals and medication schedules under the guidance of healthcare professionals.

Certain specialized diets, while not universally applicable, have garnered attention for their potential benefits in managing Parkinson's symptoms. The Mediterranean diet, renowned for its emphasis on fruits, vegetables, whole grains, and healthy fats, aligns with the nutritional principles beneficial for Parkinson's. Studies suggest that this diet may offer neuroprotective effects and contribute to improved cognitive function.

Similarly, the Ketogenic diet, characterized by low-carbohydrate and high-fat intake, has been explored for its potential impact on motor symptoms in Parkinson's. While research in this area is ongoing, early findings indicate promising avenues for further investigation into the role of dietary patterns in mitigating Parkinson's progression.

Gastrointestinal (GI) symptoms, such as constipation and dysphagia, are common challenges in Parkinson's. Dietary modifications, including increased fiber intake from fruits, vegetables, and whole grains, can contribute to regular bowel movements. Adequate fluid intake and mindful chewing also support optimal digestion and help address swallowing difficulties.

Beyond the physiological aspects, diet holds profound implications for emotional well-being. The act of preparing and sharing meals fosters social connections, combating the potential isolation often experienced by individuals with Parkinson's. A diet rich in nutrient-dense foods contributes to sustained energy levels, potentially alleviating fatigue—a prevalent symptom in Parkinson's.

While the significance of diet in Parkinson's is evident, it is essential to acknowledge the individualized nature of dietary needs. Parkinson's manifests uniquely in each individual, demanding a tailored approach that considers personal preferences, tolerances, and potential interactions with medications.

Challenges may arise, particularly in the context of altered taste perceptions, difficulties with chewing and swallowing, and fluctuations in appetite. Collaborative efforts between individuals with Parkinson's, caregivers, and healthcare professionals become paramount in devising flexible dietary plans that accommodate evolving needs and address potential barriers.

As our understanding of Parkinson's continues to evolve, ongoing research endeavors explore the dynamic relationship between diet and the intricacies of the disease. Investigations into the impact of specific nutrients, dietary patterns, and the gut-brain axis open new frontiers, offering the promise of innovative approaches for managing symptoms and potentially modifying the course of Parkinson's.

In conclusion, the importance of diet in Parkinson's extends far beyond the realm of mere sustenance. It emerges as a powerful ally in promoting overall health, supporting cognitive function, and potentially influencing the trajectory of Parkinson's disease. In the collaborative efforts of individuals, caregivers, and healthcare professionals, dietary choices become a cornerstone for empowerment—a means of nourishing not only the body but also the mind and spirit in the face of Parkinson's complex challenges.

Chapter One
What is Parkinson's Disease

Parkinson's Disease (PD) stands as a formidable adversary in the realm of neurological disorders, impacting millions of lives globally. First identified and meticulously described by Dr. James Parkinson in 1817, this chronic and progressive condition manifests primarily in the disruption of motor functions, setting in motion a complex interplay of symptoms that gradually erode the ability to move with ease and precision.

At its core, Parkinson's disease is characterized by the degeneration of nerve cells within the brain, particularly those responsible for producing dopamine—an essential neurotransmitter facilitating communication between nerve cells. The decline in dopamine levels leads to a cascade of motor symptoms that define the Parkinsonian experience.

One of the hallmark signs of Parkinson's is tremors, involuntary rhythmic shaking that commonly affects the hands but can extend to the arms, legs, jaw, or head. This physical tremor, however, is just the tip of the iceberg. The insidious progression of the disease introduces a range of motor challenges, including bradykinesia, a pervasive slowness of movement that impedes the initiation and completion of tasks. Rigidity, marked by stiffness in the limbs and trunk, adds to the physical burden, while postural instability amplifies the risk of falls, contributing to the overall complexity of living with Parkinson's.

Beyond the realm of motor functions, Parkinson's extends its reach into non-motor domains, affecting cognition, emotions, and sleep. Cognitive changes, including memory deficits and difficulties with attention, often accompany the motor symptoms. Emotional and psychological well-being also bear the brunt of the disease, with individuals experiencing heightened vulnerability to depression, anxiety, and mood fluctuations. Sleep disturbances, such as insomnia and restless legs, further compound the challenges faced by those navigating life with Parkinson's.

The causes of Parkinson's remain elusive, with a complex interplay of genetic and environmental factors implicated in its onset. While advancing age is a significant risk factor, Parkinson's can affect individuals at various stages of life. Diagnosis hinges on a combination of clinical evaluation and, in some cases, specialized imaging tests. Early detection holds paramount importance, allowing for the implementation of interventions and strategies aimed at managing symptoms and slowing the progression of the disease.

Current therapeutic approaches for Parkinson's encompass a multifaceted toolkit. Medications designed to replace or mimic dopamine aid in alleviating motor symptoms, while physical and occupational therapies provide avenues for maintaining mobility and enhancing daily living skills. In advanced cases, surgical interventions, such as deep brain stimulation (DBS), may be considered to manage symptoms and improve quality of life.

Living with Parkinson's is a journey fraught with challenges, not only for the individuals directly affected but also for their families and support networks. The intricate interplay of physical and cognitive symptoms underscores the need for a comprehensive, multidisciplinary approach to care. Ongoing research endeavors seek to unravel the mysteries of Parkinson's disease, with the ultimate goal of developing novel therapeutic interventions and, ideally, disease-modifying treatments.

In the face of this complex and evolving landscape, increased awareness and understanding emerge as crucial pillars of support. By fostering a collective consciousness about Parkinson's disease, we pave the way for a more empathetic and informed society—one that stands united in the pursuit of improved outcomes and an enhanced quality of life for those touched by this neurological challenge.

Early Signs of Parkinson

Parkinson's Disease (PD), a progressive neurodegenerative disorder, often begins its subtle intrusion long before the characteristic motor symptoms take center stage. Understanding and identifying the early signs of Parkinson's can be a pivotal step in early diagnosis and intervention, offering individuals and healthcare professionals a window of opportunity to implement strategies for better management.

While Parkinson's is conventionally associated with tremors, the initial whispers of the disease may manifest in less conspicuous ways. One of the early harbingers is a change in handwriting, often referred to as micrographia. Individuals may notice a gradual shrinking of their handwriting, with letters becoming smaller and more cramped. This seemingly innocuous shift can be an early indicator of the motor challenges that will later unfold.

Subtle changes in facial expression, known as facial masking, may also emerge in the early stages. The natural animation of the face diminishes, and individuals may appear less expressive or demonstrate a reduced range of facial movements. This diminution in facial expressivity can precede more overt motor symptoms, offering a subtle but important cue to those attuned to the nuances of Parkinson's.

Moreover, individuals in the early stages of Parkinson's may experience a decrease in their sense of smell, a phenomenon known as anosmia. While changes in the olfactory sense can be attributed to various factors, including aging, the specific association with Parkinson's becomes apparent when coupled with other emerging symptoms.

Changes in sleep patterns may also mark the early stages of Parkinson's. Individuals may find themselves grappling with disrupted sleep, experiencing difficulties falling asleep or staying asleep throughout the night. Restless leg syndrome, characterized by an irresistible urge to move the legs, particularly during periods of inactivity, can also emerge as a precursor to more overt motor symptoms.

In the realm of subtle motor changes, individuals may notice a decreased arm swing while walking or a general feeling of stiffness and mild discomfort in their limbs. These early motor alterations may be subtle and easily attributed to aging or other benign causes, making them challenging to distinguish in isolation.

It is crucial to note that the presence of one or more of these early signs does not definitively point to Parkinson's. Many conditions can mimic these symptoms, and a comprehensive medical evaluation by a healthcare professional is essential for an accurate diagnosis. Neurologists often rely on a combination of clinical history, physical examination, and sometimes specialized imaging tests to confirm the presence of Parkinson's.

Recognizing the early signs of Parkinson's disease is an evolving landscape, and ongoing research continues to unveil additional markers that may aid in early detection. The importance of vigilance and awareness in the face of subtle changes cannot be overstated, as early diagnosis opens the door to timely interventions, symptom management, and the potential to enhance the quality of life for those navigating the complexities of Parkinson's.

Causes of Parkinson's Disease

Parkinson's Disease (PD) stands as a testament to the intricate interplay of genetic and environmental factors, converging to unravel the delicate balance within the brain's neural circuits. While the precise etiology of Parkinson's remains elusive, decades of research have provided invaluable insights into the complex web of elements that contribute to the onset and progression of this neurodegenerative disorder.

At its core, Parkinson's is characterized by the degeneration of dopaminergic neurons in a region of the brain known as the substantia nigra. Dopamine, a neurotransmitter crucial for facilitating

smooth and coordinated movements, becomes deficient as these neurons succumb to degeneration. The question of what triggers this degenerative process has fueled extensive scientific inquiry.

Genetic predisposition emerges as a notable factor in the quest to unravel the causes of Parkinson's. While the majority of cases are considered sporadic, meaning they occur without a clear familial pattern, a subset of individuals has a familial form of the disease. Mutations in specific genes, such as LRRK2, PARK2, and SNCA, have been identified in familial cases and are associated with an increased risk of developing Parkinson's. The intricate dance of genetic influences offers a glimpse into the hereditary aspects of this complex condition.

Environmental factors add another layer of complexity to the causative landscape of Parkinson's. Exposure to certain toxins and chemicals has been implicated as potential contributors. Pesticides, for instance, have been studied extensively in this context, with agricultural workers and those living in rural areas exhibiting higher incidences of Parkinson's. Other environmental factors, such as head injuries, may also play a role in triggering the disease, although the mechanisms linking trauma to Parkinson's remain the subject of ongoing research.

Age, too, stands as a significant factor, with the risk of Parkinson's increasing as individuals grow older. The aging process itself may contribute to the cumulative impact of genetic and environmental factors, creating an environment ripe for the initiation of neurodegenerative processes.

Inflammation within the brain has also captured the attention of researchers studying the causes of Parkinson's. Chronic neuroinflammation is believed to play a role in the degeneration of dopaminergic neurons. The immune system, in its misguided attempt to protect the brain, may inadvertently contribute to the damage observed in Parkinson's patients.

The emerging field of gut-brain axis research has introduced yet another dimension to our understanding of Parkinson's etiology. The gastrointestinal system, once considered a mere bystander, is now recognized as a potential player in the disease's development. The aggregation of abnormal proteins, such as alpha-synuclein, which is a hallmark of Parkinson's, may begin in the gut and subsequently travel to the brain, influencing the onset of the disease.

As our knowledge of Parkinson's causes continues to evolve, it is increasingly evident that this is a multifactorial puzzle, with genetic predisposition, environmental exposures, aging, inflammation, and the intricate relationship between the gut and the brain all contributing to the complex tapestry of Parkinson's disease. The ongoing quest for a comprehensive understanding of these causes not only deepens our appreciation of the disease but also holds the promise of unveiling novel therapeutic targets and strategies for intervention, bringing us closer to a future where Parkinson's is not only understood but effectively managed and, ultimately, prevented.

Stages of Parkinson's Disease

Parkinson's Disease (PD) unfolds as a progressive journey, marked by distinct stages that characterize the evolving nature of this neurodegenerative disorder. From the initial subtle tremors to the more pervasive challenges in mobility and daily functioning, each stage presents a unique set of complexities for individuals grappling with Parkinson's and their caregivers.

The early stages of Parkinson's often begin imperceptibly, with subtle signs that may be attributed to aging or other benign factors. These may include a slight tremor in the hands, changes in handwriting, or a reduction in facial expressivity. At this juncture, known as Stage 1, individuals typically maintain a high degree of independence in their daily activities, and the symptoms may not significantly interfere with their quality of life.

As Parkinson's progresses to Stage 2, the motor symptoms become more pronounced. Bradykinesia, or slowness of movement, becomes evident, impacting the execution of everyday tasks. Rigidity, a stiffness in the limbs and trunk, contributes to a sense of physical discomfort. Despite these challenges, individuals in Stage 2 can still manage daily activities independently, although with increased effort and a growing awareness of their evolving limitations.

Stage 3 marks a pivotal juncture in the Parkinsonian journey. Balance becomes a significant concern, and postural instability increases the risk of falls. While individuals may still maintain a level of independence, the progression of symptoms begins to necessitate more comprehensive management strategies. Mobility becomes more challenging, and the need for support during certain activities becomes apparent.

Advancing to Stage 4, the impact of Parkinson's on daily life intensifies. Individuals may require assistance with various activities, and the ability to live independently becomes increasingly compromised. Despite these challenges, many individuals in Stage 4 can still stand and walk without assistance, though with notable difficulty. The fluctuations in motor function become more apparent, and the need for a supportive caregiving network becomes paramount.

The final stage, Stage 5, represents the most advanced and debilitating phase of Parkinson's disease. Individuals at this stage often experience severe motor impairments, rendering them largely incapable of independent movement. The ability to stand or walk is severely compromised, and individuals may require a wheelchair or other forms of assistance for mobility. Non-motor symptoms, including cognitive decline and emotional challenges, may also be more pronounced in Stage 5.

It is crucial to recognize that the progression through these stages is highly individualized, and not all individuals with Parkinson's will follow the same trajectory. Factors such as age, overall health, and the specific manifestations of the disease contribute to the variability in how Parkinson's unfolds in each person.

Understanding the stages of Parkinson's disease is not only vital for individuals and their families but also for healthcare professionals. This awareness informs the development of tailored treatment plans and support strategies that adapt to the evolving needs of individuals as they traverse the complex landscape of Parkinson's. As research continues to shed light on the intricacies of the disease, the hope persists for interventions that not only manage symptoms but potentially modify the course of Parkinson's, offering a brighter outlook for those navigating its challenging stages.

Diagnosis of Parkinson's Disease

Parkinson's Disease (PD) is a complex neurodegenerative disorder that demands a nuanced and thorough approach to diagnosis. While there is currently no definitive test for Parkinson's, skilled healthcare professionals employ a combination of clinical assessments, medical history analysis, and, in some cases, specialized imaging techniques to unravel the intricate tapestry of symptoms and confirm the presence of the disease.

Clinical Assessment and Symptom Recognition: The Art of Observation

The diagnosis of Parkinson's often begins with the astute observations of healthcare professionals who are trained to recognize the hallmark motor symptoms associated with the disease. Tremors, bradykinesia (slowness of movement), rigidity, and postural instability are the cardinal features that form the foundation of the clinical assessment.

Tremors, typically manifested as a rhythmic shaking, are often the most recognizable symptom. However, it is crucial to note that not all tremors are indicative of Parkinson's, and the specific characteristics, such as a resting tremor in the hands, can be significant in distinguishing Parkinson's-related tremors from other causes.

Bradykinesia, or the slowing down of voluntary movements, may be observed in everyday activities. This can manifest as a reduced arm swing while walking, difficulty initiating movements, or a general sense of sluggishness in daily tasks.

Rigidity, characterized by stiffness in the limbs and trunk, is another key motor symptom. When a healthcare professional gently moves a patient's limbs through their range of motion, resistance due to rigidity becomes apparent.

Postural instability, the tendency to lose balance and coordination, is a crucial aspect of Parkinson's diagnosis, especially in later stages. Individuals may find it challenging to maintain an upright posture and may be more prone to falls.

Beyond these motor symptoms, clinicians also pay close attention to non-motor manifestations. Changes in handwriting, known as micrographia, reduced facial expressivity (facial masking), and alterations in speech patterns may provide additional clues.

Medical History: Unraveling the Personal Narrative

The patient's medical history serves as a vital companion to the clinical assessment. Understanding the onset and progression of symptoms, as well as any relevant family history, allows healthcare professionals to piece together a comprehensive picture of the individual's Parkinsonian journey.

Patients are often queried about the timeline of symptom development, noting when they first noticed changes in movement, coordination, or other aspects of daily living. Additionally, any family history of neurodegenerative disorders is explored, as certain genetic factors can contribute to an increased risk of developing Parkinson's.

Medication history is also scrutinized, as certain drugs or their interactions may mimic Parkinsonian symptoms or exacerbate existing ones. A meticulous review of the patient's current medications and any recent changes can offer valuable insights.

The Role of Specialized Imaging: Peering Inside the Brain

While clinical assessment and medical history lay a strong foundation, specialized imaging techniques can provide a more in-depth look at the brain and its structural and functional integrity. These imaging modalities do not serve as standalone diagnostic tools but can corroborate clinical observations and help rule out other potential causes of symptoms.

Magnetic Resonance Imaging (MRI): A Detailed Portrait

MRI scans offer detailed images of the brain's structure, allowing clinicians to rule out other conditions that might be causing the observed symptoms. These images can reveal any abnormalities, such as tumors or strokes, that may present with similar symptoms to Parkinson's.

DaTscan: Illuminating Dopamine Levels

DaTscan is a nuclear medicine imaging technique that provides insights into dopamine levels in the brain. This scan involves injecting a small amount of a radioactive substance into the bloodstream, which binds to dopamine transporters. The distribution of this substance in the brain can help assess the integrity of dopamine-producing neurons.

While DaTscan is not necessary for every Parkinson's diagnosis, it can be particularly useful in cases where clinical features are ambiguous, and there is a need for further confirmation. It is worth noting that DaTscan does not distinguish between different types of parkinsonism but rather helps confirm the presence of dopaminergic deficits.

Cerebrospinal Fluid Analysis: Exploring Biomarkers

Analyzing cerebrospinal fluid can provide additional insights into the biochemical changes associated with Parkinson's disease. Elevated levels of specific proteins, such as alpha-synuclein, in the cerebrospinal fluid may suggest the presence of Parkinson's. This diagnostic approach is not as commonly employed as clinical assessments or imaging due to the invasiveness of the procedure and the availability of other diagnostic tools.

Challenges and Evolving Landscape:

Despite the progress in diagnostic methodologies, Parkinson's disease diagnosis remains a challenging endeavor. The variability in symptoms among individuals, the lack of a definitive biomarker, and the overlap of symptoms with other neurodegenerative conditions contribute to the complexity.

Moreover, the early stages of Parkinson's can be particularly elusive, with symptoms presenting subtly and often being attributed to normal aging or other benign causes. This delayed recognition poses challenges for timely intervention and the implementation of supportive strategies.

The evolving landscape of Parkinson's research brings hope for more precise and accessible diagnostic tools. Ongoing studies explore the potential of various biomarkers, such as specific proteins in blood samples, that could streamline the diagnostic process and enhance the accuracy of early detection.

Conclusion: A Holistic Approach to Diagnosis

In conclusion, the diagnosis of Parkinson's disease is a multifaceted journey that blends the art of clinical observation, the insight gained from medical history, and the precision of specialized imaging. The collaborative efforts of neurologists, movement disorder specialists, and other healthcare professionals are essential in navigating the complexities of Parkinson's diagnosis.

While there is no cure for Parkinson's, an early and accurate diagnosis empowers individuals and their healthcare teams to implement tailored strategies for symptom management and lifestyle adjustments. It also opens avenues for participation in clinical trials and the exploration of emerging therapeutic interventions aimed at slowing the progression of the disease.

As our understanding of Parkinson's continues to deepen, the diagnostic landscape is poised for evolution. Research endeavors and technological advancements hold the promise of refining diagnostic precision, ultimately enhancing the lives of those affected by Parkinson's through earlier intervention and more targeted therapeutic strategies.

Treatments for Parkinson's Disease

As our understanding of Parkinson's has deepened, so too has the spectrum of available treatments. From pharmaceutical interventions to surgical procedures, physical and occupational therapies to emerging technologies, a comprehensive approach is essential in tailoring treatments to address the diverse needs of those navigating the complexities of Parkinson's.

Pharmacological Cornerstones: Managing Motor and Non-Motor Symptoms

Pharmacological interventions form the backbone of Parkinson's disease management, primarily focused on alleviating motor symptoms by addressing the underlying deficiency of dopamine in the brain. Levodopa, often combined with carbidopa to enhance its effectiveness, remains a cornerstone medication. As a precursor to dopamine, levodopa aims to replenish the depleted neurotransmitter, mitigating the impact of motor symptoms such as tremors, rigidity, and bradykinesia.

In addition to levodopa, dopamine agonists mimic the action of dopamine in the brain, providing an alternative or complementary approach to managing symptoms. These medications include pramipexole, ropinirole, and rotigotine, offering a range of options for individuals based on their specific needs and responses.

Anticholinergic medications, such as trihexyphenidyl and benztropine, may be prescribed to address tremors and rigidity by modulating the balance between dopamine and acetylcholine, another neurotransmitter.

Catechol-O-methyltransferase (COMT) inhibitors, including entacapone and tolcapone, extend the duration of levodopa's effectiveness by preventing its breakdown in the body.

While these medications focus primarily on motor symptoms, Parkinson's encompasses a broader spectrum of challenges, including cognitive changes, emotional fluctuations, and autonomic dysfunction. Medications such as rivastigmine may be prescribed to address cognitive decline, while selective serotonin reuptake inhibitors (SSRIs) and tricyclic antidepressants target mood disorders often associated with Parkinson's.

As the disease progresses, individuals may experience motor fluctuations and dyskinesias—uncontrolled, involuntary movements induced by long-term levodopa use. To address these complications, healthcare professionals may implement advanced medication strategies, including adjusting dosages, incorporating different formulations, or considering continuous infusions via devices like duodenal pumps.

Navigating the Spectrum of Non-Motor Symptoms: Beyond Dopaminergic Therapies

Recognizing the impact of non-motor symptoms in Parkinson's is integral to comprehensive care. Depression, anxiety, sleep disturbances, and autonomic dysfunction often coexist with motor challenges, significantly influencing an individual's quality of life. Addressing these non-motor symptoms necessitates a nuanced therapeutic approach.

Psychotropic medications, including selective serotonin and norepinephrine reuptake inhibitors (SSRIs and SNRIs), may be prescribed to manage mood disorders. The use of sedative medications, such as benzodiazepines, may be considered to address sleep disturbances.

For autonomic dysfunction, medications targeting blood pressure regulation, such as fludrocortisone or midodrine, may be employed. Additionally, medications addressing gastrointestinal symptoms, such as constipation, are often part of the treatment plan.

Physical exercise, recognized for its broad-ranging benefits, serves as a non-pharmacological intervention that positively influences both motor and non-motor symptoms. Incorporating regular exercise into daily routines can enhance mobility, balance, and overall well-being.

The Promise of Surgical Interventions: Deep Brain Stimulation (DBS)

For individuals facing challenges with medication management or experiencing motor fluctuations and dyskinesias, surgical interventions may provide a transformative avenue. Deep

Brain Stimulation (DBS), a surgical procedure approved for use in Parkinson's, involves implanting electrodes into specific regions of the brain, typically the subthalamic nucleus or globus pallidus. These electrodes are connected to a stimulator device placed beneath the skin, akin to a pacemaker.

DBS modulates abnormal neuronal activity, effectively regulating motor symptoms and reducing the fluctuations associated with levodopa use. The procedure is not a cure for Parkinson's but offers a valuable tool in managing symptoms and enhancing quality of life.

While DBS has proven effective for many, careful patient selection and comprehensive evaluation are essential. The decision to undergo DBS is often collaborative, involving neurologists, neurosurgeons, and individuals with Parkinson's, taking into account factors such as disease stage, medication responsiveness, and overall health.

Rehabilitative Approaches: Physical and Occupational Therapies

Physical and occupational therapies play integral roles in the holistic management of Parkinson's. These rehabilitative approaches aim to enhance mobility, functionality, and independence, addressing both motor and non-motor aspects of the disease.

Physical therapy, tailored to individual needs, focuses on exercises that improve strength, flexibility, and balance. Gait training and functional mobility exercises aim to mitigate the risk of falls, a common concern in Parkinson's.

Occupational therapy is designed to assist individuals in performing activities of daily living (ADLs) and adapting to any physical limitations. Therapists work collaboratively with individuals to develop strategies and employ assistive devices that enhance autonomy and quality of life.

Speech therapy, often overlooked but crucial, addresses communication challenges that can arise due to changes in voice volume, articulation, and facial expressivity. Therapists employ exercises and techniques to improve vocal control and clarity, facilitating effective communication.

Emerging Technologies: Harnessing Innovation for Parkinson's Care

The landscape of Parkinson's care continues to evolve with the integration of innovative technologies. Wearable devices, such as smartwatches, provide continuous monitoring of motor symptoms, offering real-time data that can inform treatment adjustments. These devices not only aid in symptom management but also empower individuals to actively engage in their care.

Telemedicine, especially relevant in the context of global health challenges, facilitates remote consultations, enabling individuals with Parkinson's to access specialized care from the comfort of their homes. Tele-rehabilitation programs extend therapeutic interventions, allowing individuals to participate in physical and occupational therapy remotely.

Virtual reality (VR) and gaming technologies introduce a novel dimension to rehabilitative interventions. These immersive experiences engage individuals in therapeutic exercises, making rehabilitation more interactive and enjoyable.

Nutritional Interventions: The Role of Diet in Parkinson's Management

Dietary considerations extend beyond the realm of sustenance, emerging as a potential modulator of Parkinson's symptoms. While not a standalone treatment, a balanced and nutrient-dense diet contributes to overall well-being. The potential impact of certain diets, such as the Mediterranean or Ketogenic diets, on symptom management is an area of ongoing research.

Nutritional interventions also address common challenges, including constipation and swallowing difficulties. Modifications to dietary fiber intake, fluid consistency, and meal textures can enhance gastrointestinal function and support optimal nutrition.

Mind-Body Interventions: Holistic Approaches to Well-Being

Acknowledging the interconnectedness of physical and emotional well-being, mind-body interventions assume significance in the management of Parkinson's. Practices such as yoga, tai chi, and meditation offer holistic approaches that contribute to stress reduction, improved mental health, and enhanced overall resilience.

Music and art therapies, often integrated into Parkinson's care programs, tap into creative expressions as therapeutic modalities. These approaches not only provide avenues for emotional expression but also engage cognitive and motor functions.

The Importance of Individualized Care: A Personalized Path Forward

The complexity of Parkinson's disease demands an individualized and patient-centered approach to care. Each person's experience with Parkinson's is unique, necessitating a tailored treatment plan that considers the specific constellation of symptoms, medication responses, and lifestyle factors.

Regular follow-up assessments, conducted collaboratively by neurologists, movement disorder specialists, and allied healthcare professionals, allow for ongoing adjustments to treatment plans.

As Parkinson's is a dynamic condition with evolving symptoms, this iterative approach ensures that care remains responsive to the individual's changing needs.

Challenges and Future Horizons: A Call for Continued Innovation

While advancements in Parkinson's care have transformed the landscape, challenges persist. The variability in disease manifestation, the individualized responses to medications, and the dynamic nature of symptoms underscore the need for ongoing research and innovation.

The quest for disease-modifying therapies, interventions that alter the course of Parkinson's rather than solely addressing symptoms, remains a paramount goal. Clinical trials exploring novel drugs, gene therapies, and neuroprotective agents offer hope for breakthroughs that could shape the future of Parkinson's treatment.

Additionally, addressing the disparities in access to specialized care and therapies is crucial. As the global community grapples with healthcare inequities, ensuring that individuals with Parkinson's, regardless of geographic location or socioeconomic status, can avail themselves of advancements in care is an imperative.

Conclusion: A Holistic Mosaic of Care

In conclusion, the treatments for Parkinson's disease form a comprehensive mosaic, weaving together pharmacological interventions, surgical procedures, rehabilitative approaches, emerging technologies, and lifestyle modifications. The collaborative efforts of individuals, healthcare professionals, researchers, and the broader community create a tapestry of care that extends beyond symptom management, aiming to optimize overall well-being and empower individuals to navigate the complexities of Parkinson's with resilience and dignity.

As research endeavors continue to unlock new insights and therapeutic possibilities, the horizon of Parkinson's care is poised for further transformation. The synergy of innovation, individualized care, and a holistic understanding of Parkinson's positions the community on a path toward a future where the impact of the disease is not only managed but, ultimately, where breakthroughs in treatment and prevention bring forth a brighter tomorrow for those affected by Parkinson's.

Chapter Two

Nutritional Guidelines for Parkinson's Patients

Nutrition plays a crucial role in the comprehensive management of Parkinson's, influencing not only physical health but also potentially impacting cognitive function, medication efficacy, and overall well-being. As individuals navigate the complexities of Parkinson's, understanding and implementing appropriate nutritional guidelines become integral components in promoting optimal health and quality of life.

Dietary Considerations for Parkinson's Patients

1. Balanced Nutrition: The Foundation of Well-Being

A balanced and nutritious diet serves as the cornerstone for individuals with Parkinson's. Essential macronutrients, including carbohydrates, proteins, and fats, provide the energy required for daily activities. Whole grains, lean proteins, and healthy fats contribute to sustained energy levels and support overall health.

Emphasis on a varied and colorful array of fruits and vegetables introduces essential vitamins, minerals, and antioxidants. These nutrients not only nourish the body but also play a potential role in mitigating oxidative stress—a factor implicated in Parkinson's progression.

2. Protein Management: Striking the Right Balance

Protein consumption requires careful consideration for individuals with Parkinson's, especially those taking levodopa, a primary medication for managing motor symptoms. Protein intake can influence the absorption of levodopa, potentially impacting its effectiveness. While protein is an essential component of a balanced diet, strategic planning of meals and medication schedules, in consultation with healthcare professionals, helps optimize treatment outcomes.

3. Hydration: A Fundamental Pillar of Health

Adequate hydration is fundamental for everyone, and it holds particular significance for individuals with Parkinson's. Proper fluid intake supports overall health, aids in medication absorption, and addresses common issues such as constipation—a prevalent concern in Parkinson's. Individuals are encouraged to maintain a consistent and sufficient fluid intake, adapting it to their specific needs and considering factors such as medication schedules.

Nutritional Strategies for Specific Symptoms

1. Constipation Management: Fiber and Hydration

Constipation is a common challenge in Parkinson's, necessitating specific nutritional strategies. Increasing dietary fiber through whole grains, fruits, and vegetables promotes regular bowel movements. Adequate hydration complements fiber intake, facilitating optimal digestion and addressing constipation. Individual tolerance to dietary fiber varies, and adjustments should be made based on personal needs and responses.

2. Swallowing Difficulties: Texture Modifications

Swallowing difficulties, known as dysphagia, may arise in the course of Parkinson's. Modifying food textures to match individual capabilities can enhance safety and ease of swallowing. Soft or pureed foods, as well as thickened liquids, may be recommended by speech therapists or healthcare professionals. Texture modifications aim to prevent choking and aspiration, promoting a safe and enjoyable eating experience.

3. Weight Management: Addressing Changes in Appetite

Weight changes, including unintentional weight loss or gain, are considerations in Parkinson's. Changes in appetite, alterations in taste perception, and the energy expenditure associated with motor symptoms contribute to these shifts. Individualized dietary plans, developed in collaboration with healthcare professionals, address nutritional needs while managing weight fluctuations. Regular monitoring and adjustments ensure that nutritional goals align with overall health objectives.

Potential Benefits of Specific Diets

1. Mediterranean Diet: A Holistic Approach

The Mediterranean diet, characterized by an emphasis on fruits, vegetables, whole grains, and healthy fats, aligns with nutritional principles beneficial for Parkinson's. Rich in antioxidants and anti-inflammatory compounds, this diet potentially contributes to overall well-being. While not a cure for Parkinson's, the Mediterranean diet offers a holistic approach to supporting health and has been associated with cognitive benefits.

2. Ketogenic Diet: Exploring Neuroprotective Effects

The Ketogenic diet, known for its low-carbohydrate and high-fat composition, has garnered attention for its potential neuroprotective effects. Research in this area is ongoing, with early findings suggesting that the Ketogenic diet may influence motor symptoms and offer therapeutic benefits. However, the implementation of specialized diets should be approached cautiously, with careful consideration of individual health profiles and consultation with healthcare professionals.

Supplementation Considerations

1. Vitamin D and Calcium: Bone Health

Individuals with Parkinson's may be at an increased risk of bone health issues, partly due to reduced exposure to sunlight and potential mobility challenges. Supplementation with vitamin D and calcium may be recommended to support bone health. Healthcare professionals assess individual needs and guide appropriate supplementation based on nutritional status and lifestyle factors.

2. Omega-3 Fatty Acids: Cognitive Support

Omega-3 fatty acids, found in fish, flaxseeds, and walnuts, are associated with cognitive benefits. While research on the specific impact of omega-3 fatty acids in Parkinson's is ongoing, incorporating sources of these essential fats into the diet may contribute to overall cognitive health.

3. B Vitamins: Energy Metabolism

B vitamins, including B6, B12, and folate, play crucial roles in energy metabolism and neurological function. Individuals with Parkinson's may have altered absorption of these vitamins, warranting consideration of supplementation. Healthcare professionals assess nutritional status and recommend supplementation as needed to address potential deficiencies.

Holistic Approaches: Mindful Eating and Emotional Well-Being

1. Mindful Eating: Enhancing the Dining Experience

Mindful eating practices encourage a present and intentional approach to meals, fostering a deeper connection with the dining experience. Techniques such as savoring flavors, paying attention to hunger and fullness cues, and creating a pleasant dining environment contribute to an enjoyable and mindful eating experience.

2. Emotional Well-Being: Nurturing the Mind-Body Connection

The connection between emotional well-being and nutrition is profound. Addressing the psychological dimensions of Parkinson's, including stress, anxiety, and depression, involves a holistic approach. Nutrient-dense foods, coupled with mindful eating practices, contribute to emotional resilience and overall mental health. Support from mental health professionals, support groups, and holistic wellness strategies complements nutritional guidelines, nurturing the mind-body connection.

Challenges and Individual Variability: Tailoring Nutritional Guidelines

Recognizing the individual variability in nutritional needs and responses is paramount. Parkinson's manifests uniquely in each person, demanding personalized nutritional guidelines that consider specific symptoms, medication regimens, and lifestyle factors. Challenges may arise, including altered taste perceptions, difficulties with chewing and swallowing, and fluctuations in appetite. Collaborative efforts between individuals, caregivers, and healthcare professionals become pivotal in devising flexible nutritional plans that accommodate evolving needs and address potential barriers.

Future Directions and Research Horizons

Ongoing research endeavors explore the dynamic interplay between nutrition and Parkinson's disease. Investigations into the potential impact of specific nutrients, dietary patterns, and gut-brain interactions offer new frontiers in understanding how nutrition influences the trajectory of Parkinson's. The quest for biomarkers and personalized nutrition approaches holds promise for tailoring dietary interventions based on individual profiles and optimizing outcomes.

Conclusion: Empowering Through Nutrition

In conclusion, nutritional guidelines for individuals with Parkinson's disease extend beyond mere sustenance, emerging as a powerful tool in promoting overall health and well-being. A balanced and individualized approach to nutrition, encompassing dietary considerations, supplementation strategies, and mindful eating practices, contributes to the holistic management of Parkinson's.

Empowering individuals with Parkinson's to make informed dietary choices, in collaboration with healthcare professionals, not only addresses specific symptoms and challenges but also fosters a sense of agency and control in the face of a complex and progressive condition. As the landscape of Parkinson's care evolves, the integration of personalized and evidence-based nutritional guidelines becomes integral to optimizing health outcomes and enhancing the quality of life for those affected by Parkinson's.

Key Nutrients for Parkinson's Patients

While no specific diet can cure Parkinson's, a well-balanced and nutrient-rich intake is vital for managing symptoms, supporting overall health, and potentially influencing the course of the disease. In this exploration of key nutrients for individuals with Parkinson's, we delve into the roles of various vitamins, minerals, antioxidants, and other essential compounds that contribute to the holistic well-being of those navigating the challenges of Parkinson's.

1. Vitamin D: Beyond Bone Health

Vitamin D is often associated with bone health, but its significance extends far beyond calcium metabolism. Individuals with Parkinson's are at an increased risk of vitamin D deficiency due to factors such as limited sun exposure and potential mobility challenges. Adequate vitamin D levels are crucial for overall health and may contribute to cognitive function.

Research suggests that vitamin D receptors are present in the substantia nigra, a region of the brain affected by Parkinson's pathology. While the exact relationship between vitamin D and Parkinson's is complex and requires further investigation, maintaining optimal vitamin D levels through a combination of sunlight exposure and, when necessary, supplementation, is considered a prudent aspect of nutritional support.

2. Omega-3 Fatty Acids: Brain and Heart Health

Omega-3 fatty acids, including eicosapentaenoic acid (EPA) and docosahexaenoic acid (DHA), are essential for brain health and have anti-inflammatory properties. Found in fatty fish, flaxseeds, chia seeds, and walnuts, these fatty acids may play a role in supporting cognitive function and potentially mitigating neuroinflammation associated with Parkinson's.

While research on the specific impact of omega-3 fatty acids in Parkinson's is ongoing, incorporating sources of these essential fats into the diet contributes to overall cardiovascular health and may have broader implications for neurological well-being.

3. B Vitamins: Neurological Function and Energy Metabolism

The B-vitamin group, including B6, B12, and folate, is integral to neurological function and energy metabolism. Individuals with Parkinson's may experience altered absorption of these vitamins, potentially leading to deficiencies. These vitamins contribute to the synthesis of neurotransmitters, including dopamine, and play crucial roles in maintaining cognitive health.

B12 deficiency, in particular, has been associated with neurological symptoms, and supplementation may be recommended for individuals with Parkinson's, especially those following a vegetarian or vegan diet. Folate, found in green leafy vegetables and legumes, is essential for DNA synthesis and repair.

4. Antioxidants: Guarding Against Oxidative Stress

Oxidative stress, characterized by an imbalance between free radicals and antioxidants, is implicated in the neurodegenerative processes of Parkinson's. Antioxidants neutralize free radicals, potentially offering a protective effect on neurons. Key antioxidants include:

- Vitamin C: Abundant in citrus fruits, berries, and vegetables, vitamin C supports the immune system and acts as a potent antioxidant.

- Vitamin E: Found in nuts, seeds, and vegetable oils, vitamin E contributes to cellular health and may have neuroprotective effects.

- Selenium: A trace element with antioxidant properties, selenium is present in foods like nuts, seeds, and seafood.

- Polyphenols: Abundant in fruits, vegetables, tea, and red wine, polyphenols possess antioxidant and anti-inflammatory properties.

Incorporating a variety of antioxidant-rich foods into the diet provides a diverse array of these protective compounds, potentially mitigating the impact of oxidative stress in Parkinson's.

5. Vitamin K: Bone Health and Potential Neuroprotective Effects

Vitamin K is essential for blood clotting and bone health. Emerging research suggests that vitamin K may have neuroprotective effects and could influence brain health. Leafy green vegetables, such as kale and spinach, are rich sources of vitamin K. While more research is needed to establish a definitive link between vitamin K and Parkinson's, ensuring an adequate intake of this vitamin contributes to overall health.

6. Iron: Considerations for Medication Absorption

Iron plays a crucial role in oxygen transport and energy metabolism. However, iron intake may require attention, as high levels of dietary iron can potentially interfere with the absorption of levodopa, a primary medication for managing motor symptoms in Parkinson's. Individuals are advised to maintain a balanced iron intake, and consultation with healthcare professionals can guide adjustments based on individual needs.

7. Magnesium: Muscle Function and Neurological Support

Magnesium is essential for muscle function, nerve transmission, and energy production. While magnesium deficiency is not a direct cause of Parkinson's, maintaining optimal levels is vital for overall health. Magnesium-rich foods include nuts, seeds, whole grains, and leafy green vegetables. Ensuring an adequate intake of magnesium supports muscle and neurological function.

8. Zinc: Immune Function and Wound Healing

Zinc is integral to immune function, wound healing, and DNA synthesis. While the relationship between zinc and Parkinson's is complex, zinc deficiency can impact overall health. Dietary sources of zinc include meat, dairy, nuts, and legumes. Maintaining a balanced intake of zinc supports immune function and general well-being.

9. Coenzyme Q10: Mitochondrial Support

Coenzyme Q10 (CoQ10) is a compound with antioxidant properties that plays a role in mitochondrial function—the energy-producing powerhouse of cells. Some studies suggest that CoQ10 supplementation may have potential benefits in Parkinson's by supporting mitochondrial health. However, further research is needed to establish the efficacy of CoQ10 as part of Parkinson's management.

10. Protein: Strategic Consumption for Medication Management

Protein is a fundamental component of the diet, providing essential amino acids necessary for bodily functions. However, protein consumption requires strategic consideration for individuals with Parkinson's, particularly those taking levodopa. High-protein meals can interfere with the absorption of levodopa, potentially affecting its effectiveness. Collaborative discussions with healthcare professionals guide individuals in optimizing protein intake while managing medication schedules.

Conclusion: A Holistic Nutritional Approach to Parkinson's Care

In conclusion, a holistic approach to nutritional support for individuals with Parkinson's encompasses a diverse array of key nutrients that contribute to overall health and well-being. While no single nutrient or diet can serve as a cure for Parkinson's, a balanced intake of essential vitamins, minerals, antioxidants, and other compounds supports neurological function, mitigates oxidative stress, and potentially influences the course of the disease.

Individualized nutritional plans, developed in collaboration with healthcare professionals, address specific needs, dietary preferences, and potential interactions with medications. Regular monitoring and adjustments ensure that nutritional goals align with overall health objectives, fostering a sense of empowerment and well-being for individuals navigating the complexities of Parkinson's.

As ongoing research endeavors explore the dynamic interplay between nutrition and Parkinson's, the landscape of nutritional guidelines is poised for further refinement. The integration of personalized and evidence-based nutritional support emerges as a vital component in optimizing health outcomes and enhancing the quality of life for those affected by Parkinson's.

Chapter Three
Parkinson's-Friendly Foods

While there is no specific diet that can cure Parkinson's, certain foods can be particularly beneficial in managing symptoms, supporting overall health, and optimizing the quality of life for individuals navigating this complex condition. In this exploration of Parkinson's-friendly foods, we delve into the nutritional considerations, dietary patterns, and specific food choices that contribute to holistic well-being for those affected by Parkinson's.

Balanced Nutrition: A Foundation for Parkinson's Care

1. Fruits and Vegetables: Antioxidant Powerhouses

A colorful array of fruits and vegetables constitutes a cornerstone of a Parkinson's-friendly diet. Rich in vitamins, minerals, and antioxidants, these foods contribute to overall health and potentially mitigate the impact of oxidative stress—a factor implicated in the progression of Parkinson's.

- Berries: Blueberries, strawberries, and raspberries are packed with antioxidants and anti-inflammatory compounds, offering potential neuroprotective effects.

- Leafy Greens: Spinach, kale, and Swiss chard are rich in folate, vitamin K, and iron, supporting cognitive function and overall well-being.

- Colorful Vegetables: Bell peppers, tomatoes, and carrots provide a diverse range of nutrients, including vitamins A and C, and contribute to antioxidant defenses.

2. Whole Grains: Sustained Energy and Fiber

Whole grains form a vital component of a Parkinson's-friendly diet, providing sustained energy and essential dietary fiber. Fiber supports digestive health, helps regulate blood sugar levels, and contributes to overall satiety.

- Quinoa: A complete protein source, quinoa is rich in fiber, magnesium, and iron, supporting muscle function and overall well-being.

- Oats: Oats are a good source of soluble fiber, promoting heart health and providing a steady release of energy.

- Brown Rice: Brown rice is a whole grain with a range of nutrients, including B vitamins and manganese, supporting energy metabolism.

3. Lean Proteins: Essential Amino Acids

Protein is a fundamental building block for bodily functions, and incorporating lean sources into the diet is crucial for individuals with Parkinson's. Essential amino acids derived from protein contribute to neurotransmitter synthesis and overall muscle health.

- Chicken: Skinless, lean chicken breast is a versatile and high-quality protein source.

- Fish: Fatty fish, such as salmon, mackerel, and trout, provide omega-3 fatty acids and protein, supporting brain health.

- Legumes: Beans, lentils, and chickpeas are plant-based protein sources rich in fiber, vitamins, and minerals.

Strategic Considerations for Protein Intake

1. Timing of Protein Consumption

Given the potential interaction between protein and levodopa absorption—the primary medication for managing motor symptoms in Parkinson's—strategic timing of protein intake is important. Spreading protein consumption throughout the day, with a focus on lower-protein meals during levodopa absorption times, can help optimize medication effectiveness.

2. Variety in Protein Sources

Diversifying protein sources ensures a comprehensive intake of essential amino acids and other nutrients. Including both animal and plant-based proteins contributes to overall dietary balance and supports muscle health.

Healthy Fats: Omega-3s and Monounsaturated Fats

1. Fatty Fish: Omega-3 Fatty Acids

Fatty fish, such as salmon, tuna, and sardines, are rich in omega-3 fatty acids. These essential fats have anti-inflammatory properties and may contribute to cognitive health.

2. Avocado: Monounsaturated Fats

Avocado is a nutrient-dense fruit rich in monounsaturated fats. These heart-healthy fats provide a source of sustained energy and contribute to overall well-being.

Fluids: Hydration and Beyond

1. Water: Optimal Hydration

Adequate hydration is crucial for everyone, and individuals with Parkinson's are no exception. Proper fluid intake supports overall health, aids in medication absorption, and helps prevent issues such as constipation—a common concern in Parkinson's.

   - Herbal Teas: Caffeine-sensitive individuals may find herbal teas, such as chamomile or peppermint, to be soothing and hydrating alternatives.

   - Infused Water: Adding natural flavors to water with slices of fruits or herbs enhances hydration and adds a refreshing twist.

Mindful Eating: Enhancing the Dining Experience

1. Texture Modifications

Individuals with Parkinson's, especially those experiencing swallowing difficulties, may benefit from texture modifications. Soft or pureed foods, as well as thickened liquids, enhance safety and ease of swallowing.

2. Adaptive Utensils

Using adaptive utensils, such as weighted or ergonomic options, can assist individuals with motor challenges in maintaining independence during meals.

Foods with Potential Benefits in Parkinson's Management

1. Turmeric: Curcumin's Anti-Inflammatory Properties

Turmeric, and its active compound curcumin, has anti-inflammatory and antioxidant properties. While more research is needed, incorporating turmeric into meals may offer potential benefits in managing inflammation associated with Parkinson's.

2. Green Tea: Polyphenols for Brain Health

Green tea contains polyphenols, which have antioxidant and neuroprotective properties. While research on green tea and Parkinson's is ongoing, moderate consumption may contribute to overall brain health.

Nutritional Considerations for Medication Interactions

Considering the interaction between levodopa and dietary proteins, individuals are advised to work with healthcare professionals to find a personalized balance that optimizes medication effectiveness while ensuring adequate protein intake.

Challenges and Individual Variability: Tailoring the Diet

Parkinson's manifests uniquely in each individual, demanding a tailored approach to the diet that considers personal preferences, tolerances, and potential interactions with medications. Collaborative efforts between individuals, caregivers, and healthcare professionals are crucial in devising flexible dietary plans that accommodate evolving needs and address potential barriers.

Conclusion: Empowering Through Nutrition

In conclusion, Parkinson's-friendly foods form a diverse and nourishing palette that contributes to the holistic well-being of individuals affected by Parkinson's. While there is no one-size-fits-all approach, incorporating a variety of nutrient-dense foods, strategic protein considerations, and mindful eating practices empowers individuals to optimize their nutritional intake in the face of the challenges posed by Parkinson's.

As research endeavors continue to uncover the intricate connections between nutrition and Parkinson's, the landscape of dietary recommendations is poised for further refinement. The integration of personalized and evidence-based nutritional strategies becomes pivotal in optimizing health outcomes, supporting cognitive function, and enhancing the quality of life for those navigating the complexities of Parkinson's. By fostering a sense of agency and well-being through informed dietary choices, individuals with Parkinson's can embark on a journey towards holistic health and resilience.

Recipes and Meal Ideas

A Parkinson's diagnosis introduces a unique set of challenges, but maintaining a nutritious and enjoyable diet is crucial for overall well-being. A carefully crafted meal plan can address specific needs associated with Parkinson's Disease (PD), such as potential interactions with medications, swallowing difficulties, and the need for sustained energy. In this comprehensive guide, we explore a variety of recipes and meal ideas tailored to the needs of Parkinson's patients, with a focus on enhancing nutrition, managing symptoms, and promoting an enjoyable dining experience.

Breakfast Ideas

1. Nutrient-Rich Smoothie Bowl:

- Ingredients: Berries (blueberries, strawberries), banana, Greek yogurt, almond milk, chia seeds, spinach.

- Method: Blend berries, banana, Greek yogurt, and almond milk. Pour into a bowl and top with chia seeds and fresh spinach for added nutrients.

2. Oatmeal with Nuts and Fruit:

- Ingredients: Rolled oats, almond milk, sliced almonds, walnuts, banana, honey.

- Method: Cook rolled oats with almond milk. Top with sliced almonds, walnuts, and banana slices. Drizzle with honey for sweetness.

3. Protein-Packed Breakfast Burrito:

- Ingredients: Whole-grain tortilla, scrambled eggs, black beans, diced tomatoes, avocado, salsa.

- Method: Fill a whole-grain tortilla with scrambled eggs, black beans, diced tomatoes, and avocado. Top with salsa for added flavor.

4. Chia Seed Pudding:

- Ingredients: Chia seeds, almond milk, vanilla extract, fresh fruit (berries or sliced kiwi).

- Method: Mix chia seeds with almond milk and vanilla extract. Refrigerate overnight. Top with fresh fruit before serving.

Lunch and Dinner Recipes

1. Salmon and Quinoa Salad:

- Ingredients: Grilled salmon, quinoa, mixed greens, cherry tomatoes, cucumber, lemon vinaigrette.

- Method: Place grilled salmon on a bed of cooked quinoa and mixed greens. Add cherry tomatoes and sliced cucumber. Drizzle with a lemon vinaigrette.

2. Chicken and Vegetable Stir-Fry:

- Ingredients: Stir-fry chicken strips, broccoli, bell peppers, snap peas, low-sodium soy sauce.

- Method: Stir-fry chicken and vegetables in a pan with low-sodium soy sauce. Serve over brown rice.

3. Vegetarian Lentil Soup:

- Ingredients: Lentils, vegetable broth, carrots, celery, onion, garlic, cumin, coriander.

- Method: Cook lentils in vegetable broth with carrots, celery, onion, and garlic. Season with cumin and coriander for a flavorful soup.

4. Spinach and Feta Stuffed Chicken Breast:

   - Ingredients: Chicken breast, fresh spinach, feta cheese, garlic, olive oil.

   - Method: Butterfly chicken breast and stuff with fresh spinach and feta. Drizzle with olive oil and bake until cooked through.

Side Dishes and Snacks

1. Baked Sweet Potato Fries:

   - Ingredients: Sweet potatoes, olive oil, paprika, salt.

   - Method: Cut sweet potatoes into fries, toss with olive oil, paprika, and salt. Bake until crispy.

2. Hummus and Veggie Platter:

   - Ingredients: Hummus, carrot sticks, cucumber slices, bell pepper strips.

   - Method: Arrange a variety of colorful vegetables around a bowl of hummus for a nutritious and satisfying snack.

3. Greek Yogurt Parfait:

   - Ingredients: Greek yogurt, granola, mixed berries, honey.

   - Method: Layer Greek yogurt with granola and mixed berries. Drizzle with honey for a delicious parfait.

4. Edamame with Sea Salt:

   - Ingredients: Edamame (soybeans), sea salt.

   - Method: Steam edamame and sprinkle with sea salt for a protein-rich and easy-to-eat snack.

Dessert Ideas

1. Frozen Banana Bites:

   - Ingredients: Banana slices, peanut butter, dark chocolate.

   - Method: Spread peanut butter on banana slices and freeze. Dip in melted dark chocolate for a sweet and satisfying treat.

2. Chia Seed Chocolate Pudding:

   - Ingredients: Chia seeds, almond milk, cocoa powder, maple syrup.

- Method: Mix chia seeds with almond milk, cocoa powder, and maple syrup. Refrigerate until set.

3. Baked Apple with Cinnamon:

   - Ingredients: Apple, cinnamon, honey.

   - Method: Core an apple and sprinkle with cinnamon. Bake until tender. Drizzle with honey before serving.

4. Berries and Cream:

   - Ingredients: Mixed berries, Greek yogurt, honey.

   - Method: Combine mixed berries with a dollop of Greek yogurt. Drizzle with honey for a simple and nutritious dessert.

Beverage Options

1. Green Tea with Ginger:

   - Ingredients: Green tea bags, fresh ginger slices, honey.

   - Method: Brew green tea with fresh ginger slices. Sweeten with honey to taste.

2. Berry and Spinach Smoothie:

   - Ingredients: Mixed berries, fresh spinach, almond milk, protein powder (optional).

   - Method: Blend mixed berries, fresh spinach, almond milk, and protein powder for a nutrient-packed smoothie.

3. Turmeric Latte:

   - Ingredients: Turmeric powder, almond milk, cinnamon, honey.

   - Method: Warm almond milk with turmeric, cinnamon, and honey for a soothing turmeric latte.

4. Hydrating Coconut Water with Mint:

   - Ingredients: Coconut water, fresh mint leaves.

   - Method: Infuse coconut water with fresh mint leaves for a refreshing and hydrating beverage.

Considerations for Parkinson's Patients

1. Texture Modifications:

- For individuals with swallowing difficulties, consider modifying the texture of foods, such as pureeing vegetables into soups or choosing softer alternatives.

2. Adaptive Utensils:

- Use adaptive utensils, such as weighted or ergonomic options, to assist with ease of use during meals.

3. Protein Timing:

- Consider spreading protein intake throughout the day and aligning protein-rich meals with times when levodopa absorption is not a concern.

4. Nutrient Density:

- Prioritize nutrient-dense foods to ensure that meals are packed with essential vitamins, minerals, and antioxidants.

5. Individual Preferences:

- Tailor recipes to individual preferences and dietary restrictions, making adjustments based on taste preferences and tolerances.

Conclusion: Crafting a Nutrient-Rich Culinary Journey

In conclusion, crafting a nutrient-rich and enjoyable culinary journey for individuals with Parkinson's involves a thoughtful selection of ingredients, consideration of potential challenges, and an understanding of personal preferences. The recipes and meal ideas provided here offer a diverse array of options to enhance nutrition, manage symptoms, and promote an overall positive dining experience.

As with any dietary plan, it is essential to collaborate with healthcare professionals, including dietitians and neurologists, to ensure that meal choices align with individual health needs and medication regimens. Empowering individuals with Parkinson's to enjoy delicious and nourishing meals not only contributes to their physical well-being but also enhances their quality of life and

the joy derived from the act of dining. By embracing creativity and flexibility in the kitchen, individuals with Parkinson's can embark on a culinary journey that supports their health and brings a sense of satisfaction and pleasure to their daily lives.

Practical Meal Planning Strategies

Meal planning is a crucial aspect of managing Parkinson's Disease (PD), as it plays a significant role in supporting overall health, optimizing medication effectiveness, and addressing potential challenges related to nutrition. Individuals with Parkinson's, along with their caregivers, can benefit from practical meal planning strategies that take into account their unique needs and preferences. In this comprehensive guide, we explore practical approaches to meal planning, focusing on nutrient-dense choices, timing considerations for medications, and the importance of adaptability to enhance the dining experience for those navigating Parkinson's.

Foundations of Parkinson's-Friendly Meal Planning

1. Nutrient-Dense Choices: Building a Balanced Plate

- Colorful Fruits and Vegetables: Incorporate a variety of colorful fruits and vegetables into meals. These are rich in essential vitamins, minerals, and antioxidants, contributing to overall health.

- Whole Grains: Choose whole grains, such as quinoa, brown rice, and oats, for sustained energy and fiber. These grains provide essential nutrients supporting overall well-being.

- Lean Proteins: Include lean protein sources like poultry, fish, beans, and legumes. Protein is vital for muscle health and overall bodily functions.

- Healthy Fats: Opt for sources of healthy fats, such as avocados, nuts, and olive oil. These contribute to brain health and provide sustained energy.

- Dairy or Alternatives: Select dairy or dairy alternatives fortified with calcium and vitamin D to support bone health.

2. Strategic Considerations for Protein Intake

- Timing of Protein Consumption: Given the potential interaction between protein and levodopa absorption, distribute protein intake evenly throughout the day. Consider consuming lower-protein meals during levodopa absorption times.

- Protein Variety: Diversify protein sources to ensure a comprehensive intake of essential amino acids. Include both animal and plant-based proteins in the diet for balance.

3. Hydration: A Fundamental Aspect of Nutrition

- Adequate Water Intake: Stay well-hydrated to support overall health. Proper fluid intake is crucial for medication absorption and helps prevent issues such as constipation, a common concern in Parkinson's.

- Herbal Teas and Infusions: Consider herbal teas like chamomile or peppermint, which are hydrating and may have soothing effects. Infuse water with natural flavors using fruits or herbs.

Adapting Meals to Parkinson's Challenges

1. Texture Modifications for Swallowing Difficulties

- Soft and Pureed Options: For individuals with swallowing difficulties, modify textures by incorporating soft or pureed foods. Soups, stews, and blended options can enhance safety and ease of swallowing.

- Nutrient-Rich Smoothies: Create nutrient-dense smoothies using fruits, vegetables, yogurt, and protein powder. Smoothies provide a convenient way to pack in essential nutrients.

2. Adaptive Utensils for Motor Challenges

- Weighted and Ergonomic Utensils: Utilize adaptive utensils with weighted or ergonomic designs to assist individuals with motor challenges during meals. These tools enhance independence and ease of use.

- Plate Guards and Non-Skid Mats: Implement plate guards to prevent spills and non-skid mats to stabilize plates and utensils. These adaptations enhance the overall dining experience.

3. Mindful Eating Practices

- Slow and Conscious Eating: Encourage slow and conscious eating to enhance the dining experience. This practice can aid in better digestion and allow individuals to savor the flavors of their meals.

- Reduced Distractions: Minimize distractions during meals to promote focused and enjoyable eating. Create a calm and pleasant environment to enhance the overall dining experience.

Meal Planning Throughout the Day

1. Breakfast Ideas for Sustained Energy

- Protein-Packed Breakfast: Include protein-rich options such as eggs, Greek yogurt, or lean meats to provide sustained energy throughout the morning.

- Whole Grain Choices: Opt for whole grain cereals, oats, or whole grain toast to provide fiber and essential nutrients.

- Fruit and Nut Parfait: Create a parfait with layers of Greek yogurt, fresh fruits, and nuts for a nutrient-dense and flavorful breakfast.

2. Lunch and Dinner: Balanced and Nourishing Meal

- Salmon and Quinoa Bowl: Incorporate grilled salmon, quinoa, and a variety of vegetables for a well-balanced and nutrient-rich bowl.

- Vegetarian Stir-Fry: Prepare a colorful stir-fry with a mix of vegetables, tofu, and a flavorful sauce. Serve over brown rice for added fiber.

- Spinach and Feta Stuffed Chicken: Stuff chicken breasts with spinach and feta for a protein-packed and delicious dinner option.

- Lentil Soup: Prepare a hearty lentil soup with vegetables for a plant-based protein source and a variety of nutrients.

3. Side Dishes and Snacks: Supporting Nutrient Intake

- Greek Yogurt with Berries: Combine Greek yogurt with fresh berries for a satisfying and protein-rich snack.

- Baked Sweet Potato Fries: Bake sweet potato fries for a nutritious alternative to traditional fries, providing vitamins and fiber.

- Hummus and Vegetable Platter: Pair hummus with carrot sticks, cucumber slices, and bell pepper strips for a tasty and nutrient-packed snack.

- Edamame with Sea Salt: Steam edamame and sprinkle with sea salt for a protein-rich and satisfying snack.

4. Desserts: Balanced and Flavorful Options

- Frozen Banana Bites: Dip banana slices in peanut butter and dark chocolate for a sweet and nutritious dessert.

- Chia Seed Chocolate Pudding: Create a chia seed pudding using almond milk, cocoa powder, and maple syrup for a satisfying chocolate treat.

- Baked Apple with Cinnamon: Bake apples with a sprinkle of cinnamon for a warm and naturally sweet dessert.

- Berries and Cream: Combine mixed berries with Greek yogurt for a refreshing and healthful dessert option.

Beverages: Supporting Hydration and Enjoyment

1. Herbal Teas and Infusions:

   - Chamomile Tea: Known for its calming properties, chamomile tea can be a soothing choice.

   - Peppermint Tea: Peppermint tea may aid digestion and provide a refreshing flavor.

2. Smoothies and Nutrient-Rich Drinks:

   - Berry and Spinach Smoothie: Blend mixed berries, fresh spinach, almond milk, and protein powder for a nutrient-packed smoothie.

   - Turmeric Latte: Warm almond milk with turmeric, cinnamon, and honey for a soothing and anti-inflammatory beverage.

3. Hydrating Options:

   - Infused Water: Enhance water with natural flavors by adding slices of fruits or herbs.

   - Coconut Water with Mint: Infuse coconut water with fresh mint leaves for a hydrating and refreshing drink.

Considerations for Medication Timing and Food

1. Levodopa Timing and Protein Interaction:

   - Balanced Protein Intake: Distribute protein intake evenly throughout the day, considering levodopa absorption times.

   - Collaborate with Healthcare Professionals: Work with healthcare professionals to develop an individualized protein intake plan that aligns with medication schedules.

2. Meal Timing and Medication Administration:

   - Consistent Schedules: Maintain consistent meal and medication schedules to support the effectiveness of Parkinson's medications.

   - Planning for Off Periods: Anticipate "off" periods and have easily digestible snacks or meals available during these times.

Adaptability and Flexibility in Meal Planning

1. Exploring New Ingredients and Recipes:

  - Diverse Culinary Exploration: Embrace a variety of cuisines and ingredients to keep meals interesting and flavorful.

  - Incorporating Superfoods: Explore the inclusion of superfoods such as turmeric, ginger, and dark leafy greens for their potential anti-inflammatory and health-promoting properties.

2. Tailoring to Personal Preferences and Tolerances:

  - Individualized Approaches: Recognize individual preferences and dietary tolerances when planning meals. Tailor recipes to align with personal tastes and comfort levels.

3. Seeking Support and Inspiration:

  - Community and Support Groups: Engage with community or online support groups to share meal planning tips, recipes, and experiences.

  - Cookbooks and Resources: Explore Parkinson's-friendly cookbooks and nutritional resources for inspiration and guidance.

Conclusion: Empowering Through Nutrition

In conclusion, practical meal planning strategies for Parkinson's aim to empower individuals to make informed choices that support overall health, medication effectiveness, and an enjoyable dining experience. By incorporating nutrient-dense foods, adapting meals to address specific challenges, and considering the timing of medications, individuals with Parkinson's can enhance their well-being and maintain a positive relationship with food.

Moreover, the adaptability and flexibility in meal planning allow for a personalized approach that aligns with individual preferences and tolerances. Seeking support from healthcare professionals, dietitians, and the Parkinson's community can provide valuable insights and encouragement on this culinary journey.

Through thoughtful and intentional meal planning, individuals with Parkinson's can nourish both their bodies and minds, fostering a sense of empowerment and well-being in their daily lives.

Chapter Four
Foods to Limit or Avoid

Parkinson's Disease (PD) is a complex neurodegenerative disorder that necessitates careful consideration of dietary choices. While there is no specific diet that can cure Parkinson's, certain foods may have an impact on symptoms, medication effectiveness, and overall well-being. In this comprehensive guide, we explore foods that individuals with Parkinson's may consider limiting or avoiding, taking into account potential interactions with medications, symptom management, and overall health.

1. High-Protein Foods: Balancing Intake with Medication

One of the primary considerations for individuals with Parkinson's is the interaction between protein intake and levodopa absorption—the main medication for managing motor symptoms. Levodopa competes with dietary proteins for absorption in the small intestine, potentially affecting its effectiveness. Therefore, while protein is an essential component of a healthy diet, strategic planning of protein intake is crucial.

Foods to Limit:

- Red meat

- Poultry

- Fish

- Dairy products

- Legumes

Strategies:

- Distribute protein intake evenly throughout the day.

- Consider lower-protein meals during levodopa absorption times.

- Collaborate with healthcare professionals to determine an individualized protein intake plan.

2. Foods High in Saturated and Trans Fats: Impact on Cardiovascular Health

A diet high in saturated and trans fats is associated with an increased risk of cardiovascular diseases. Individuals with Parkinson's should be mindful of heart health, as cardiovascular issues can coexist with the disease.

Foods to Limit or Avoid:

- Fried foods

- Processed snacks

- Full-fat dairy products

- Fatty cuts of meat

- Commercially baked goods

Strategies:

- Choose lean protein sources.

- Opt for healthy fats, such as those found in avocados, nuts, and olive oil.

- Prioritize whole foods over processed options.

3. Excessive Sodium: Implications for Blood Pressure and Medication Interaction

High sodium intake can contribute to elevated blood pressure, and some individuals with Parkinson's may be more susceptible to orthostatic hypotension—a drop in blood pressure upon standing. Additionally, certain medications may increase the risk of dehydration, making sodium management crucial.

Foods to Limit:

- Processed foods

- Canned soups

- Pickled and preserved foods

- Deli meats

- Restaurant/fast-food meals

Strategies:

- Choose fresh, whole foods.

- Cook meals at home to control salt content.

- Use herbs and spices for flavor instead of excessive salt.

4. Refined Sugars and Simple Carbohydrates: Impact on Blood Sugar Levels

A diet high in refined sugars and simple carbohydrates can lead to fluctuations in blood sugar levels. Individuals with Parkinson's may benefit from stable blood sugar levels to support energy levels and overall health.

Foods to Limit or Avoid:

- Sugary snacks and desserts

- Soda and sugary drinks

- White bread

- White rice

- Highly processed cereals

Strategies:

- Choose whole grains over refined grains.

- Opt for natural sources of sweetness, such as fruits.

- Monitor carbohydrate intake to maintain stable blood sugar levels.

5. Oxalate-Rich Foods: Consideration for Kidney Stones

Some individuals with Parkinson's may have an increased risk of kidney stones. While dietary factors are just one aspect of kidney stone prevention, limiting certain oxalate-rich foods may be beneficial.

Foods to Limit:

- Spinach

- Rhubarb

- Beets

- Nuts and seeds

- Chocolate

Strategies:

- Consume oxalate-rich foods in moderation.

- Stay hydrated to support kidney health.

- Discuss dietary considerations with healthcare professionals.

6. Caffeine: Balance for Medication Sensitivity

Caffeine sensitivity can be heightened in individuals with Parkinson's, and it may interact with certain medications. While moderate caffeine consumption is generally considered safe, individuals should be mindful of its potential effects.

Foods to Limit:

- Coffee

- Tea

- Chocolate

- Energy drinks

Strategies:

- Monitor individual tolerance to caffeine.

- Consider consuming caffeine earlier in the day to minimize potential interference with sleep.

- Collaborate with healthcare professionals to find an appropriate balance.

7. Aspartame: Potential Sensitivity

Aspartame, an artificial sweetener, has been associated with potential sensitivity in some individuals with Parkinson's. While research in this area is ongoing, those who experience sensitivity may choose to limit their aspartame intake.

Foods to Limit:

- Diet sodas

- Sugar-free gum

- Sugar-free desserts

Strategies:

- Choose alternatives sweetened with natural sugars or explore other sweeteners.

- Pay attention to individual reactions and consult healthcare professionals.

8. Alcohol: Consideration for Medication Interaction and Balance

While moderate alcohol consumption is generally considered acceptable for many individuals, those with Parkinson's should be mindful of potential interactions with medications and the impact on balance and coordination.

Foods to Limit:

- Alcoholic beverages

Strategies:

- If consuming alcohol, do so in moderation.

- Be aware of potential interactions with Parkinson's medications.

- Discuss alcohol consumption with healthcare professionals.

Conclusion: Personalized Approaches to Dietary Choices

In conclusion, navigating nutrition in Parkinson's involves personalized approaches to dietary choices. While there are general guidelines on foods to limit or avoid, it is crucial to recognize the individual variability in responses to different foods and the potential impact on symptom management and overall health.

Collaboration with healthcare professionals, including neurologists and dietitians, is essential to tailor dietary recommendations to individual needs and considerations. Understanding the potential interactions between certain foods and Parkinson's medications, as well as addressing specific symptoms or health concerns, empowers individuals to make informed choices that support their well-being.

Ultimately, the goal is to strike a balance between managing symptoms, supporting overall health, and promoting an enjoyable and sustainable approach to eating. By adopting a mindful and personalized approach to nutrition, individuals with Parkinson's can navigate their dietary journey with a sense of empowerment and well-being.

Managing Medication Interactions

Medications play a crucial role in alleviating symptoms and improving the quality of life for individuals with Parkinson's. However, the effectiveness of these medications can be influenced by various factors, including diet. In this comprehensive guide, we explore the intricate relationship between Parkinson's medications and food, offering insights into how individuals can navigate their dietary choices to optimize treatment outcomes.

Understanding Parkinson's Medications

Before delving into the specifics of medication interactions with food, it is essential to understand the common medications prescribed for Parkinson's:

1. Levodopa:

   - Levodopa is a precursor to dopamine, a neurotransmitter that is deficient in Parkinson's.

   - Commonly prescribed in combination with carbidopa to enhance its effectiveness.

   - Absorption can be influenced by dietary factors, particularly protein intake.

2. Dopamine Agonists:

   - Mimic the effects of dopamine in the brain.

   - Examples include pramipexole and ropinirole.

   - May be taken with or without food, depending on individual tolerance.

3. MAO-B Inhibitors:

   - Monoamine oxidase B (MAO-B) inhibitors, such as rasagiline and selegiline, help preserve dopamine levels.

   - Some interactions with certain foods and medications.

4. COMT Inhibitors:

- Catechol-O-methyltransferase (COMT) inhibitors, like entacapone, prolong the effects of levodopa.

- Taken with levodopa and carbidopa.

Understanding how these medications work and their potential interactions with food sets the stage for effective management and enhanced treatment outcomes.

1. Levodopa: Balancing Protein Intake

One of the primary considerations for individuals taking levodopa is the interaction with dietary proteins. Levodopa competes with amino acids for absorption in the small intestine, and high-protein meals can potentially reduce its effectiveness.

Strategies:

- Timing of Protein Intake: Distribute protein intake evenly throughout the day. Consider consuming lower-protein meals during levodopa absorption times.

- Collaboration with Healthcare Professionals: Work closely with healthcare professionals, including neurologists and dietitians, to tailor protein intake to individual needs.

- Individualized Plans: Recognize the variability in protein tolerance among individuals and create personalized dietary plans.

2. Dopamine Agonists: Considerations for Individual Tolerance

Dopamine agonists, such as pramipexole and ropinirole, may be taken with or without food, depending on individual tolerance. Some individuals may experience nausea as a side effect, and taking medications with food can help alleviate this symptom.

Strategies:

- Individualized Timing: Determine the most suitable time for medication administration with consideration for individual tolerance.

- Food as a Buffer: Taking medications with a small snack or meal can serve as a buffer, potentially reducing nausea.

- Consultation with Healthcare Professionals: Collaborate with healthcare professionals to find an optimal medication schedule that aligns with dietary preferences.

3. MAO-B Inhibitors: Managing Tyramine Interactions

MAO-B inhibitors, including rasagiline and selegiline, help preserve dopamine levels by inhibiting the enzyme monoamine oxidase B. These medications interact with foods containing tyramine, a compound that can lead to increased blood pressure.

Foods to Avoid:

- Aged cheeses

- Fermented or pickled foods

- Cured meats

- Certain alcoholic beverages

- Some soy products

Strategies:

- Dietary Restrictions: Adhere to dietary restrictions regarding tyramine-containing foods to prevent potential interactions.

- Education and Awareness: Educate individuals and caregivers about tyramine-containing foods and the importance of avoiding them.

- Monitoring Blood Pressure: Regularly monitor blood pressure, especially when initiating or adjusting MAO-B inhibitors.

4. COMT Inhibitors: Supporting Levodopa Efficacy

Catechol-O-methyltransferase (COMT) inhibitors, such as entacapone, work by prolonging the effects of levodopa. While these medications are typically taken with levodopa and carbidopa, their interactions with food are not as pronounced as with levodopa alone.

Strategies:

- Consistent Medication Timing: Take COMT inhibitors consistently with levodopa and carbidopa to support their combined effectiveness.

- Individualized Adjustments: Collaborate with healthcare professionals to make individualized adjustments to medication timing based on response and tolerability.

5. General Considerations for Medication Administration

Apart from specific interactions with certain medications, there are general considerations for optimizing the administration of Parkinson's medications in relation to food:

- Consistency is Key: Strive for consistency in medication timing to maintain stable symptom control.

- Individualized Schedules: Recognize that individual responses to medications may vary, and adjustments to medication schedules may be necessary.

- Monitoring and Communication: Regularly monitor symptoms, side effects, and overall well-being. Open communication with healthcare professionals is essential for making informed adjustments.

Food-Drug Interactions: Beyond Medications for Parkinson's

In addition to Parkinson's-specific medications, individuals may be prescribed medications for comorbidities or other health conditions. Understanding potential interactions between these medications and food is crucial for overall health and well-being.

1. Medications and Grapefruit Interaction:

   - Some medications, including certain statins and antihypertensives, can interact with grapefruit, leading to altered drug metabolism.

   - Individuals should consult with healthcare professionals to determine if grapefruit or grapefruit juice should be avoided.

2. Iron and Levodopa Interaction:

   - Iron supplements or iron-rich foods can potentially reduce the absorption of levodopa.

   - Individuals taking iron supplements or with high iron intake should separate iron consumption from levodopa administration.

Practical Tips for Managing Medication-Food Interactions

1. Keep a Medication and Food Diary:

   - Maintain a detailed diary documenting medication schedules, food intake, and symptom fluctuations.

- This diary can serve as a valuable tool during healthcare appointments and facilitate discussions with professionals.

2. Regularly Review Medications with Healthcare Professionals:

- Schedule regular reviews of medications with neurologists or movement disorder specialists.

- Discuss any changes in symptoms, side effects, or dietary preferences to make informed adjustments.

3. Collaborate with Dietitians:

- Work closely with dietitians to develop individualized dietary plans that align with medication regimens.

- Seek guidance on managing dietary restrictions, nutritional needs, and potential interactions.

4. Educate Caregivers:

- Ensure that caregivers are educated about the specific medication regimen, potential interactions, and dietary considerations.

- Foster open communication between individuals with Parkinson's, caregivers, and healthcare professionals.

5. Stay Informed About New Medications and Research:

- Stay informed about advancements in Parkinson's medications and potential interactions with food.

- Attend support groups, seminars, or educational events to stay updated on the latest research.

Conclusion: A Holistic Approach to Parkinson's Management

In conclusion, managing medication interactions with food in Parkinson's requires a holistic and individualized approach. By understanding the nuances of how different medications work and their potential interactions with dietary choices, individuals can empower themselves to optimize treatment outcomes.

Open communication with healthcare professionals, consistent monitoring of symptoms, and a collaborative effort between individuals, caregivers, and the healthcare team are pivotal in navigating the complex landscape of Parkinson's management. As research advances and new therapeutic options emerge, staying informed and adapting strategies accordingly becomes essential for fostering the best possible quality of life for individuals living with Parkinson's.

Chapter Five
Exercise and Its Role

While there is currently no cure for Parkinson's, emerging research and clinical evidence highlight the profound impact of exercise in managing symptoms, improving overall function, and potentially slowing disease progression. In this comprehensive exploration, we delve into the role of exercise as a therapeutic intervention for Parkinson's, examining its physiological mechanisms, diverse modalities, and the holistic benefits it offers to individuals navigating the complexities of this neurological condition.

Exercise and Neuroplasticity: Rewiring the Brain

Neuroplasticity, the brain's ability to adapt and reorganize itself in response to experience, forms the foundation of exercise's impact on Parkinson's. Research indicates that engaging in regular physical activity can induce neuroplastic changes that contribute to improved neural connectivity, enhanced motor learning, and potentially neuroprotective effects.

1. Promotion of Neurotrophic Factors: Exercise stimulates the production of neurotrophic factors, such as brain-derived neurotrophic factor (BDNF), which support the survival and growth of neurons. This neurotrophic support may be particularly beneficial in the context of Parkinson's, where neuronal loss is a central feature.

2. Dopaminergic System Modulation: Physical activity has been shown to modulate the dopaminergic system, potentially influencing the release and utilization of dopamine. This modulation contributes to the amelioration of motor symptoms and may impact the progression of the disease.

3. Synaptic Plasticity Enhancement: Exercise fosters synaptic plasticity, strengthening connections between neurons. This enhanced synaptic plasticity can facilitate adaptive responses to neuronal challenges, promoting resilience in the face of neurodegenerative processes.

Diverse Modalities of Exercise for Parkinson's

1. Aerobic Exercise:

 - Benefits: Aerobic exercise, such as walking, jogging, cycling, or swimming, improves cardiovascular fitness, enhances mood, and contributes to overall well-being.

 - Impact on Parkinson's Symptoms: Studies suggest that aerobic exercise may positively influence motor symptoms, including gait disturbances and bradykinesia.

2. Strength Training:

 - Benefits: Strength training, involving resistance exercises, enhances muscle strength, improves balance, and supports bone health.

 - Impact on Parkinson's Symptoms: Resistance training has been associated with improvements in muscle strength, mobility, and functional independence.

3. Balance and Flexibility Exercises:

 - Benefits: Balance and flexibility exercises, encompassing activities like tai chi, yoga, and stretching routines, enhance proprioception, posture, and range of motion.

 - Impact on Parkinson's Symptoms: These exercises contribute to improved balance, reduced risk of falls, and increased flexibility, addressing common challenges in Parkinson's.

4. Dance and Rhythmic Movements:

 - Benefits: Dance-based activities, whether structured dance classes or spontaneous movements to music, offer a dynamic and enjoyable way to engage in physical activity.

 - Impact on Parkinson's Symptoms: Dance has shown promise in addressing motor symptoms, promoting coordination, and fostering a sense of rhythm and fluidity in movements.

5. Cognitive Exercises:

- Benefits: Cognitive exercises, including dual-task activities that combine physical movement with cognitive challenges, enhance cognitive function and multitasking abilities.

- Impact on Parkinson's Symptoms: Integrating cognitive elements into exercise routines may improve cognitive performance and mitigate the impact of cognitive decline associated with Parkinson's.

6. Adaptive and Functional Exercises:

- Benefits: Adaptive exercises, tailored to individual abilities and challenges, focus on functional movements relevant to daily life.

- Impact on Parkinson's Symptoms: Functional exercises contribute to enhanced daily functioning, increased independence, and improved quality of life.

Tailoring Exercise Programs to Individual Needs

1. Assessment and Individualized Plans:

- Comprehensive Evaluation: Before initiating an exercise program, individuals with Parkinson's should undergo a comprehensive evaluation, considering their overall health, specific symptoms, and existing fitness levels.

- Collaboration with Healthcare Professionals: Collaborate with healthcare professionals, including neurologists, physical therapists, and exercise specialists, to develop individualized exercise plans.

2. Incorporating Variety and Enjoyment:

- Diverse Modalities: Include a variety of exercise modalities to address different aspects of physical health, enhance motivation, and prevent monotony.

- Incorporating Enjoyable Activities: Choose activities that individuals enjoy to foster adherence and sustained engagement in the exercise routine.

3. Adapting to Progression and Challenges:

- Regular Monitoring: Regularly monitor progress and adapt exercise routines to accommodate changes in symptoms, fitness levels, or overall health.

- Modifying Intensity and Duration: Modify the intensity and duration of exercises based on individual capabilities, ensuring a balance between challenge and safety.

4. Incorporating Social Elements:

- Group Activities: Engage in group exercise classes or activities to incorporate social elements, providing a supportive and motivating environment.

- Community Involvement: Participate in community-based exercise programs or support groups to foster a sense of camaraderie and shared experiences.

5. Home-Based Exercise Programs:

- Convenience and Accessibility: Explore home-based exercise programs, especially beneficial for individuals with mobility challenges or those who prefer the convenience of exercising at home.

- Telehealth Options: Utilize telehealth resources for virtual exercise sessions guided by professionals.

Benefits Beyond Motor Symptom Management

1. Cognitive Benefits:

- Cognitive Reserve Enhancement: Engaging in regular exercise may contribute to the building of cognitive reserve, potentially slowing cognitive decline associated with Parkinson's.

- Multitasking Improvement: Cognitive exercises that incorporate multitasking can enhance cognitive flexibility and multitasking abilities.

2. Psychosocial Well-Being:

- Mood Enhancement: Exercise has well-documented mood-enhancing effects, contributing to the alleviation of depression and anxiety commonly experienced by individuals with Parkinson's.

- Social Interaction: Group exercise activities provide opportunities for social interaction, reducing feelings of isolation and fostering a sense of community.

3. Sleep Quality Improvement:

- Regulation of Sleep Patterns: Regular exercise can contribute to the regulation of sleep patterns, potentially improving sleep quality—an important aspect of overall well-being.

4. Potential Neuroprotective Effects:

- Research Insights: Emerging research suggests that exercise may have neuroprotective effects, potentially influencing the course of Parkinson's at a cellular level.

- Animal Studies: Animal studies indicate that physical activity may promote the release of neurotrophic factors and support neuronal survival.

Addressing Common Challenges in Exercise Adherence

1. Motivational Strategies:

   - Setting Realistic Goals: Establish realistic and achievable exercise goals, recognizing individual capabilities and constraints.

   - Tracking Progress: Maintain a log of exercise sessions and progress, celebrating achievements and milestones along the way.

2. Adapting to Fluctuating Symptoms:

   - Flexible Exercise Plans: Design exercise plans that allow for flexibility to accommodate days of fluctuating symptoms or fatigue.

   - Adjusting Intensity: Modify the intensity or type of exercise based on how an individual feels on a particular day.

3. Incorporating Enjoyable Activities:

   - Personal Preferences: Tailor exercise routines to align with personal preferences, whether it's dancing, gardening, or swimming.

   - Exploring New Activities: Encourage exploration of new activities to keep the routine interesting and enjoyable.

4. Social Engagement:

   - Group Activities: Joining group exercise classes or activities provides social support and motivation.

   - Virtual Communities: Explore online platforms and virtual communities focused on Parkinson's-friendly exercises, fostering a sense of connection.

Exercise as a Collaborative Effort: The Role of Caregivers and Healthcare Professionals

1. Caregiver Involvement:

   - Support and Encouragement: Caregivers play a crucial role in providing support, encouragement, and assistance as needed.

- Participating in Activities: Caregivers can join individuals in exercise activities, creating a shared experience and promoting motivation.

2. Healthcare Professional Guidance:

- Specialized Programs: Seek guidance from healthcare professionals, including physical therapists or certified exercise specialists with expertise in Parkinson's.

- Regular Monitoring: Healthcare professionals can monitor progress, adjust exercise plans, and provide guidance on adapting to changing health conditions.

3. Interdisciplinary Approach:

- Collaboration Among Specialists: Foster collaboration among different specialists, including neurologists, physical therapists, and occupational therapists, to create a comprehensive and tailored approach to care.

Conclusion: A Dynamic Partnership Between Movement and Well-Being

In conclusion, exercise emerges as a powerful ally in the multifaceted journey of Parkinson's. Beyond its role in managing motor symptoms, exercise engages the brain's capacity for adaptation, promotes neuroplasticity, and contributes to a holistic sense of well-being. The diverse modalities of exercise cater to individual preferences and challenges, offering a personalized approach that goes beyond a one-size-fits-all paradigm.

As the landscape of Parkinson's care evolves, the integration of exercise into comprehensive management plans becomes increasingly imperative. By fostering a dynamic partnership between movement and well-being, individuals with Parkinson's, their caregivers, and healthcare

professionals can collectively harness the transformative power of exercise to enhance the quality of life and navigate the complexities of this neurological condition with resilience and empowerment.

Sleep and Stress Management

Recognizing the intricate relationship between Parkinson's, sleep quality, and stress management is crucial for optimizing overall well-being. In this comprehensive guide, we delve into the complexities of sleep in Parkinson's, explore the impact of stress on the condition, and provide practical strategies for promoting restorative sleep and managing stress.

Understanding Sleep Disturbances in Parkinson's Disease

Sleep disturbances are common in Parkinson's Disease, affecting both the quantity and quality of sleep. Individuals with Parkinson's may experience various sleep-related challenges, including insomnia, restless legs syndrome (RLS), periodic limb movements in sleep (PLMS), and rapid eye movement (REM) sleep behavior disorder. These disturbances not only contribute to daytime fatigue but can also exacerbate other Parkinson's symptoms.

1. Insomnia:

   - Difficulty Initiating or Maintaining Sleep: Individuals with Parkinson's may struggle with both falling asleep and staying asleep, leading to fragmented and insufficient sleep.

   - Contributing Factors: Factors such as motor symptoms, medication side effects, or anxiety can contribute to insomnia in Parkinson's.

2. Restless Legs Syndrome (RLS):

   - Unpleasant Sensations in the Legs: RLS is characterized by uncomfortable sensations in the legs, often described as tingling, crawling, or aching.

   - Aggravation During Rest: Symptoms typically worsen during periods of rest or inactivity, making it challenging to relax and fall asleep.

3. Periodic Limb Movements in Sleep (PLMS):

   - Involuntary Leg Movements: PLMS involves repetitive and involuntary leg movements during sleep, potentially causing disruptions in sleep architecture.

   - Associations with Daytime Fatigue: The presence of PLMS may contribute to daytime fatigue and decreased overall sleep quality.

4. REM Sleep Behavior Disorder (RBD):

   - Loss of Normal Muscle Atonia: Individuals with RBD act out their dreams due to the absence of the normal paralysis of muscles during REM sleep.

   - Safety Concerns: RBD can lead to disruptive behaviors during sleep, including kicking, punching, or falling out of bed, posing safety concerns for both individuals and their sleep partners.

The Bidirectional Relationship: Parkinson's, Sleep, and Stress

1. Impact of Parkinson's on Sleep:

  - Motor Symptoms and Sleep Disruptions: Motor symptoms, such as tremors and rigidity, can interfere with comfortable sleep positions, contributing to sleep disturbances.

  - Medication Side Effects: Certain medications prescribed for Parkinson's may have side effects that affect sleep, including insomnia, vivid dreams, or daytime sleepiness.

2. Impact of Poor Sleep on Parkinson's Symptoms:

  - Exacerbation of Motor and Non-Motor Symptoms: Inadequate or disrupted sleep can worsen motor symptoms, cognitive function, and mood in individuals with Parkinson's.

  - Reduced Coping Abilities: Sleep disturbances may compromise an individual's ability to cope with stressors, further amplifying the impact of Parkinson's on daily life.

3. Stress as a Contributing Factor:

  - Altered Neurotransmitter Balance: Stress activates the sympathetic nervous system, leading to the release of stress hormones and potentially altering the delicate balance of neurotransmitters, including dopamine, in the brain.

  - Exacerbation of Non-Motor Symptoms: Stress may exacerbate non-motor symptoms such as anxiety, depression, and cognitive impairment, contributing to sleep disturbances.

Strategies for Improving Sleep Quality in Parkinson's

1. Establishing a Consistent Sleep Routine:

  - Regular Bedtime and Wake-Up Times: Maintain a consistent sleep schedule, going to bed and waking up at the same time each day to regulate the body's internal clock.

  - Creating a Relaxing Bedtime Routine: Engage in calming activities before bedtime, such as reading, listening to soothing music, or practicing relaxation techniques.

2. Optimizing Sleep Environment:

- Comfortable Mattress and Pillows: Ensure the mattress and pillows provide adequate support and comfort for minimizing discomfort during sleep.

- Dark and Quiet Room: Create a sleep-conducive environment by minimizing light and noise in the bedroom.

3. Managing Medication Timing:

- Coordinate with Healthcare Professionals: Collaborate with healthcare professionals to optimize the timing of Parkinson's medications, considering their impact on sleep.

- Balancing Symptom Management: Balance the need for symptom management with the goal of minimizing potential sleep disruptions caused by medications.

4. Addressing Restless Legs Syndrome (RLS):

- Medication Options: Consult with healthcare providers about medications that can alleviate RLS symptoms.

- Non-Pharmacological Approaches: Consider non-pharmacological approaches, such as regular exercise and warm baths, to manage RLS symptoms.

5. Managing Periodic Limb Movements in Sleep (PLMS):

- Evaluation and Treatment: If PLMS is suspected, seek evaluation by a sleep specialist for appropriate diagnosis and potential treatment options.

- Consideration of Medications: In some cases, medications may be prescribed to manage PLMS, but the decision should be made in consultation with healthcare professionals.

6. Navigating REM Sleep Behavior Disorder (RBD):

- Safety Measures: Implement safety measures in the bedroom, such as removing potentially hazardous objects, to mitigate the risks associated with RBD.

- Consultation with Sleep Specialists: Consult with sleep specialists to explore treatment options for managing RBD and improving sleep safety.

7. Cognitive Behavioral Therapy for Insomnia (CBT-I):

- Evidence-Based Approach: CBT-I is an evidence-based therapeutic approach for treating insomnia that focuses on modifying behaviors and thoughts related to sleep.

- Individualized Sessions: Consider participating in CBT-I sessions, either in person or through telehealth, for personalized strategies to improve sleep.

8. Physical Activity and Exercise:

- Incorporating Regular Exercise: Engage in regular physical activity, incorporating both aerobic and strength-training exercises, to promote overall health and potentially improve sleep quality.

- Timing Considerations: Schedule exercise sessions earlier in the day, as late-night workouts may be stimulating and interfere with sleep.

Stress Management Strategies for Individuals with Parkinson's

1. Mindfulness and Relaxation Techniques:

- Mindfulness Meditation: Practice mindfulness meditation to cultivate present-moment awareness and reduce the impact of stressors on mental well-being.

- Deep Breathing Exercises: Incorporate deep breathing exercises, such as diaphragmatic breathing, to promote relaxation and alleviate stress.

2. Yoga and Tai Chi:

- Mind-Body Practices: Engage in mind-body practices like yoga or tai chi, which combine physical movement with mindfulness, promoting relaxation and stress reduction.

- Balance Improvement: Both yoga and tai chi can also contribute to improved balance, addressing a common concern in Parkinson's.

3. Creative Outlets and Hobbies:

- Artistic Expressstre Explore creative outlets such as painting, writing, or music to express emotions and channel stress into positive endeavors.

- Engaging in Hobbies: Pursue hobbies that bring joy and fulfillment, providing a respite from stressors associated with Parkinson's.

4. Social Support and Connection:

- Maintaining Relationships: Cultivate and maintain social connections, whether with family, friends, or support groups, to provide a network of emotional support.

- Open Communication: Share feelings and experiences with trusted individuals, fostering a sense of understanding and empathy.

5. Counseling and Psychotherapy:

- Professional Support: Consider individual or group counseling with a mental health professional experienced in working with individuals with chronic conditions.

- Cognitive-Behavioral Therapy (CBT):** CBT can be particularly beneficial for addressing stress, anxiety, and depression, offering practical coping strategies.

6. Time Management and Prioritization:

- Setting Realistic Goals: Establish realistic goals and priorities, recognizing personal capabilities and limitations.

- Effective Time Management: Develop effective time management strategies to reduce feelings of overwhelm and enhance a sense of control.

7. Adaptive Coping Mechanisms:

- Flexibility and Adaptability: Cultivate a mindset of flexibility and adaptability when facing challenges associated with Parkinson's.

- Positive Reframing: Practice reframing negative thoughts into more positive and empowering perspectives.

8. Holistic Approaches:

- Acupuncture and Massage: Explore holistic approaches, such as acupuncture or massage therapy, which may contribute to relaxation and stress reduction.

- Nutritional Support: Ensure a balanced and nutritious diet to support overall health, as nutritional choices can impact both physical and mental well-being.

Caregiver Support in Sleep and Stress Management

1. Open Communication:

- Understanding Individual Needs: Caregivers should communicate openly with individuals with Parkinson's to understand their unique sleep patterns, stressors, and preferences for support.

- Expressing Concerns: Express concerns related to sleep and stress management, fostering collaborative problem-solving.

2. Respite Care and Support Groups:

- Respite Opportunities: Seek respite care opportunities to allow caregivers periods of rest and rejuvenation.

- Participation in Support Groups: Participate in caregiver support groups to share experiences, exchange coping strategies, and access emotional support.

3. Educational Resources:

- Understanding Parkinson's Impact: Caregivers can benefit from educational resources that provide insights into how Parkinson's may affect sleep and stress levels.

- **Access to Professional Guidance:** Gain access to professional guidance, including healthcare providers and mental health professionals, for tailored advice and support.

Conclusion: A Holistic Approach to Well-Being in Parkinson's

In conclusion, the intricate interplay between Parkinson's Disease, sleep, and stress necessitates a holistic approach to well-being. By understanding the specific sleep challenges associated with Parkinson's and implementing targeted strategies, individuals can work towards achieving restorative and rejuvenating sleep. Simultaneously, stress management techniques empower individuals and caregivers to navigate the emotional complexities of living with a chronic condition.

The integration of evidence-based practices, such as cognitive-behavioral therapy for insomnia (CBT-I), mindfulness, and physical activity, forms a foundation for promoting sleep quality and stress resilience. Caregivers play a pivotal role in providing support, fostering open communication, and seeking resources to enhance the overall quality of life for individuals with Parkinson's.

As the landscape of Parkinson's care evolves, the recognition of sleep and stress as integral components of well-being becomes paramount. Through a collaborative effort between individuals, caregivers, and healthcare professionals, a comprehensive approach to sleep and stress management emerges—one that embraces the multifaceted nature of Parkinson's and nurtures serenity amidst life's challenges.

Conclusion

Success Stories: Personal Journeys with the Parkinson's Diet

In the realm of Parkinson's Disease (PD), where each day may pose unique challenges, the significance of dietary choices has garnered increasing attention. The Parkinson's Diet, often characterized by its emphasis on nutrient-dense foods, mindful eating, and personalized adaptations, has become a focal point for individuals navigating the complexities of this neurodegenerative condition. In this exploration, we delve into success stories—real, poignant narratives of individuals who have embraced and thrived on the Parkinson's Diet. These personal journeys not only illuminate the transformative power of nutrition but also serve as beacons of inspiration for those seeking ways to enhance their well-being while living with Parkinson's.

Story 1

In the beginning, many individuals with Parkinson's find themselves facing uncertainties about how dietary changes might impact their journey. The story of Alex, a 62-year-old diagnosed with Parkinson's five years ago, showcases the transformative potential of a culinary awakening.

Alex's journey with the Parkinson's Diet began when he attended a nutrition workshop tailored for those with neurodegenerative conditions. Initially skeptical, he gradually embraced the concept of using food as medicine. Alex recalls, "I was used to seeing food as merely a source of energy, but the workshop opened my eyes to the potential of food in managing Parkinson's symptoms."

With newfound enthusiasm, Alex started incorporating nutrient-dense foods into his daily meals. He adopted a colorful array of fruits and vegetables, leaned into whole grains, and explored lean protein sources. "I began to view each meal as an opportunity to nourish my body," he reflects.

Remarkably, as Alex adjusted his dietary habits, he noticed subtle improvements in his energy levels and mood. Encouraged by these positive changes, he continued to fine-tune his diet, eventually developing a personalized approach that suited his preferences and accommodated Parkinson's-specific challenges.

Story 2: The Art of Adaptation

Adapting to dietary changes can be a journey of resilience and creativity. Sarah, a 55-year-old artist diagnosed with Parkinson's, discovered the art of adaptation through her exploration of the Parkinson's Diet.

Sarah's journey began with a determination to infuse creativity into her culinary endeavors. Inspired by the vibrant hues of her paintings, she sought out colorful fruits and vegetables to elevate both the visual and nutritional appeal of her meals. "I realized that the more visually appealing my plate, the more I enjoyed my food," Sarah reflects.

However, Parkinson's presented unique challenges, including fine motor difficulties. Undeterred, Sarah embraced adaptive strategies, such as using specialized utensils and exploring new textures. "I started incorporating smoothies and soups into my diet, ensuring I still received essential nutrients without compromising on flavor," she shares.

In Sarah's story, adaptation became an art form—a testament to the resilience of the human spirit when faced with challenges. Through ingenuity and a commitment to nourishing her body, she discovered a culinary landscape that not only supported her health but also reflected her artistic ethos.

Story 3: From Challenge to Culinary Mastery

Turning dietary challenges into opportunities for culinary mastery is exemplified by James, a 68-year-old former chef who refused to let Parkinson's limit his gastronomic prowess.

Upon receiving his Parkinson's diagnosis, James experienced a period of adjustment to the motor challenges that accompanied the condition. Faced with tremors and decreased dexterity, he initially found conventional cooking methods challenging. Determined to reignite his passion for culinary excellence, James delved into the world of adaptive cooking techniques.

"I started experimenting with slow cookers and one-pot recipes," James recounts. "These methods not only made cooking more manageable for me but also enhanced the flavors of the dishes."

James's journey became a testament to the fusion of culinary expertise and adaptability. His kitchen transformed into a haven of innovation, where he discovered the nuances of Parkinson's-friendly ingredients and techniques. Through dedication and a commitment to his culinary craft, James not only overcame the challenges posed by Parkinson's but elevated his gastronomic skills to new heights.

Story 4: Shared Tables, Shared Triumphs

The communal aspect of dining takes center stage in Emily's narrative, showcasing the role of shared tables in fostering support, connection, and shared triumphs within the Parkinson's community.

Emily, a 60-year-old with Parkinson's, discovered the power of community through a Parkinson's Diet support group. "Sharing meals and experiences with others who understood the nuances of Parkinson's made a world of difference," she reflects.

The support group became a source of inspiration and shared wisdom. Members exchanged recipes, discussed dietary strategies, and celebrated each other's culinary triumphs. "We turned our gatherings into a celebration of life through food," Emily recounts.

In the shared tables of the Parkinson's community, individuals found not only nourishment for the body but also sustenance for the soul. The act of breaking bread together became a symbol of resilience, camaraderie, and shared triumphs over the challenges posed by Parkinson's.

Story 5: A Family Affair

The impact of the Parkinson's Diet extends beyond the individual diagnosed; it resonates within families, creating a ripple effect of positive change. The story of the Miller family exemplifies the transformative influence of a family-wide commitment to the Parkinson's Diet.

When Michael, the patriarch of the Miller family, was diagnosed with Parkinson's, the entire family rallied together to explore dietary strategies that could benefit him. With a shared commitment to supporting Michael's well-being, they embarked on a collective journey toward healthier eating.

"The Parkinson's Diet became a family affair," says Lisa, Michael's wife. Together, they redesigned their weekly grocery shopping, opting for fresh produce, lean proteins, and whole grains. They experimented with Parkinson's-friendly recipes, finding joy in the collaborative process of creating nourishing meals.

Remarkably, the dietary changes didn't just impact Michael; they influenced the entire family's health. "We all started feeling more energized, and the kitchen became a space for shared experiences and laughter," Lisa shares.

In the Miller family's narrative, the Parkinson's Diet became a catalyst for familial unity, well-being, and a shared commitment to thriving in the face of Parkinson's challenges.

Story 6: A Journey of Discovery

For many, embracing the Parkinson's Diet is a journey of discovery—of new tastes, textures, and the profound connection between nutrition and well-being. This theme is exemplified in the story of Maria, a 63-year-old diagnosed with Parkinson's who embarked on a journey of culinary exploration.

Maria's initial response to the Parkinson's Diet was marked by curiosity. Eager to understand the impact of specific foods on her symptoms, she began keeping a detailed food diary. "It was a journey of discovery," Maria reflects. "I started noticing patterns between certain foods and how I felt."

Through this process of self-discovery, Maria identified foods that seemed to positively influence her energy levels and mood. She gradually built a repertoire of Parkinson's-friendly recipes that aligned with her preferences and sensitivities. "It wasn't about restriction; it was about finding what made me feel good," she emphasizes.

In Maria's narrative, the Parkinson's Diet transformed from a set of guidelines into a canvas for self-exploration and empowerment. Through her culinary journey, she not only gained insights into the interplay between food and well-being but also found a sense of agency in navigating life with Parkinson's.

Chapter 7: Breaking Barriers with Bold Flavors

The Parkinson's Diet is not synonymous with blandness or monotony; rather, it is an invitation to explore a world of bold flavors and culinary creativity. The story of Raj, a 50-year-old diagnosed with early-onset Parkinson's, exemplifies how embracing diverse and robust flavors can be a catalyst for breaking dietary barriers.

Raj, a passionate food enthusiast, refused to let Parkinson's limit his palate. Instead, he saw it as an opportunity to explore a myriad of spices, herbs, and global cuisines. "I discovered that bold flavors not only made my meals more enjoyable but also brought a sense of adventure to my plate," he shares.

Raj's kitchen became a laboratory of taste, where he experimented with spices known for their potential anti-inflammatory properties. Turmeric, cumin, and ginger found their way into his recipes, creating a fusion of flavors that not only delighted his taste buds but also contributed to his well-being.

In Raj's narrative, bold flavors became a symbol of empowerment—a declaration that Parkinson's wouldn't dictate the richness and vibrancy of his culinary experiences. Through his bold culinary explorations, Raj broke down barriers and demonstrated that the Parkinson's Diet could be a journey of culinary liberation.

Story 8: Beyond the Plate—Mindful Eating and Holistic Wellness**

The Parkinson's Diet extends beyond the mere selection of foods; it encompasses the practice of mindful eating and the pursuit of holistic wellness. In the story of Elena, a 57-year-old with Parkinson's, the integration of mindful eating became a transformative aspect of her overall well-being.

Elena's journey began with a realization—food was not just fuel; it was an integral part of her self-care routine. She embraced the concept of mindful eating, savoring each bite and paying attention to the sensory experience of her meals. "Mindful eating allowed me to fully engage with the pleasure of food," she reflects.

As Elena cultivated a mindful approach to her meals, she noticed a profound impact on her digestion, mood, and overall satisfaction with her dietary choices. "I became attuned to my body's signals, making choices that truly nourished me," she shares.

Elena's story emphasizes the transformative power of mindful eating—a practice that goes beyond the plate and extends into the realms of holistic wellness. By weaving mindfulness into her culinary journey, she not only enhanced her relationship with food but also embraced a comprehensive approach to well-being.

Conclusion: A Tapestry of Inspiration

The success stories woven into the fabric of the Parkinson's Diet form a tapestry of inspiration— a testament to the resilience, creativity, and transformative power of individuals facing the challenges of Parkinson's Disease. Through culinary awakenings, adaptations, shared triumphs, family unity, self-discovery, bold flavors, and mindful eating, these individuals have embraced a holistic approach to well-being.

As we reflect on these narratives, it becomes evident that the Parkinson's Diet is not a one-size-fits-all prescription but a dynamic and personalized journey. It is a journey of exploration, empowerment, and the recognition that food can be a source of joy, vitality, and connection.

The stories of Alex, Sarah, James, Emily, the Miller family, Maria, Raj, and Elena serve as beacons of hope for those navigating Parkinson's. They invite individuals to reimagine their relationship with food, to view the kitchen as a canvas for creativity, and to recognize the profound impact of dietary choices on the intricate tapestry of Parkinson's wellness.

In each narrative, the Parkinson's Diet emerges not as a constraint but as a pathway to empowerment—a culinary journey that transcends limitations and embraces the richness of life. As individuals with Parkinson's and their families embark on their own culinary odysseys, these success stories illuminate the way, offering inspiration, guidance, and the promise that, even in the face of challenges, triumphs on the plate are within reach.

Common Questions and Answers

The Parkinson's Diet, a nuanced and evolving approach to nutrition, has sparked numerous questions among individuals living with Parkinson's Disease (PD) and their caregivers. As the awareness of the impact of diet on Parkinson's symptoms grows, so does the curiosity and inquiry about best practices, dietary modifications, and the role of nutrition in overall well-being. In this comprehensive exploration, we delve into common questions surrounding the Parkinson's Diet, providing informed answers to guide individuals on their journey towards better health and vitality.

Question 1: What is the Parkinson's Diet, and how does it differ from a standard diet?

The Parkinson's Diet is a specialized approach to nutrition that focuses on optimizing well-being and managing symptoms associated with Parkinson's Disease. Unlike a standard diet, the Parkinson's Diet tailors food choices to address the unique challenges posed by the condition. Emphasis is placed on nutrient-dense foods, anti-inflammatory components, and mindful eating practices. This personalized approach aims to support physical health, enhance energy levels, and potentially alleviate specific Parkinson's symptoms.

Question 2: Are there specific foods that individuals with Parkinson's should include in their diet?

Yes, several foods are commonly recommended for individuals with Parkinson's due to their potential benefits. These include:

- Fruits and Vegetables: Rich in antioxidants and vitamins, fruits and vegetables are cornerstones of the Parkinson's Diet. Berries, leafy greens, and colorful produce are particularly encouraged.

- Whole Grains: Whole grains provide fiber and essential nutrients. Options such as brown rice, quinoa, and oats are favorable choices.

- Lean Proteins: Including lean protein sources like poultry, fish, beans, and legumes helps support muscle health without excessive saturated fat intake.

- Omega-3 Fatty Acids: Found in fatty fish, flaxseeds, and walnuts, omega-3 fatty acids may have anti-inflammatory properties and could benefit brain health.

- Turmeric: Known for its anti-inflammatory properties, turmeric is a spice often recommended in the Parkinson's Diet.

- Green Tea: Rich in antioxidants, green tea may have neuroprotective effects and contribute to overall health.

Question 3: Are there foods that individuals with Parkinson's should avoid?

While dietary needs vary among individuals, some commonly recommended guidelines suggest limiting or avoiding certain foods, including:

- Excessive Saturated Fats: High intake of saturated fats, often found in red meat and full-fat dairy, may be associated with increased inflammation.

- Processed Foods: Highly processed foods with additives and preservatives may contribute to inflammation and are generally discouraged.

- Excessive Sugar: A diet high in refined sugars may contribute to inflammation and should be moderated.

- Artificial Sweeteners: Some individuals find that artificial sweeteners can impact their symptoms, so their consumption is often minimized.

- High-Sodium Foods: Excessive sodium intake can contribute to high blood pressure, a concern for individuals with Parkinson's, so it's advisable to limit salt intake.

Question 4: How can the Parkinson's Diet address non-motor symptoms such as depression and constipation?

The Parkinson's Diet isn't solely focused on motor symptoms; it also considers non-motor symptoms. Nutrient-dense foods and specific dietary choices may positively influence mood and gastrointestinal health:

- Omega-3 Fatty Acids: Found in fatty fish, omega-3 fatty acids may have mood-stabilizing effects and could contribute to mental well-being.

- Probiotics: Incorporating probiotic-rich foods like yogurt, kefir, and fermented vegetables may support gut health and alleviate constipation.

- Hydration: Ensuring adequate water intake is crucial for preventing dehydration and promoting digestive regularity.

- Fiber: Whole grains, fruits, and vegetables rich in fiber can aid in maintaining bowel regularity.

- Balanced Diet: A balanced and varied diet provides essential nutrients that contribute to overall well-being, potentially influencing mood and digestive health positively.

Question 5: Can dietary changes impact the effectiveness of Parkinson's medications?

It's essential for individuals with Parkinson's to coordinate any significant dietary changes with their healthcare team, especially concerning medication. Certain foods may interact with Parkinson's medications, affecting absorption or efficacy. For example:

- Protein Timing: Some individuals find that the timing of protein intake in relation to medication can influence its effectiveness. Working with healthcare professionals to establish a consistent routine is advisable.

- Iron and Levodopa: High doses of iron supplements may impact the absorption of levodopa, a common medication for Parkinson's. Managing iron intake, especially through supplements, should be discussed with healthcare providers.

- Vitamin B6: Excessive intake of vitamin B6, often found in supplements, may interfere with levodopa. Monitoring B6 intake from supplements and fortified foods is recommended.

Question 6: How can the Parkinson's Diet accommodate individuals with swallowing difficulties?

Swallowing difficulties, known as dysphagia, can be a concern in Parkinson's. The Parkinson's Diet can be adapted to address these challenges:

- Texture Modifications: Foods can be modified in texture, such as pureeing or chopping, to make them easier to swallow. This may include softer fruits, well-cooked vegetables, and ground meats.

- Hydration: Adequate hydration can aid in swallowing, so incorporating soups, smoothies, and other liquid-based options is beneficial.

- Speech and Language Therapy: Seeking guidance from a speech and language therapist can provide personalized strategies for managing dysphagia and adapting the diet accordingly.

- Nutritional Supplements: In cases where meeting nutritional needs through regular foods is challenging, healthcare professionals may recommend nutritional supplements to ensure adequate nutrient intake.

Question 7: How does the Parkinson's Diet address weight management concerns, including both weight loss and weight gain?

Weight management is a multifaceted aspect of the Parkinson's Diet, and the approach may differ based on individual needs:

- Weight Loss: For those experiencing unintentional weight loss, focusing on nutrient-dense, calorie-rich foods can be beneficial. Incorporating healthy fats, lean proteins, and frequent, smaller meals may help maintain or gain weight.

- Weight Gain: Conversely, for individuals concerned about weight gain, adopting a balanced and portion-controlled diet can be helpful. Prioritizing whole foods and incorporating regular physical activity supports overall health without promoting excess weight gain.

- Individualized Plans: Working with healthcare professionals and, if needed, consulting with a registered dietitian can help develop individualized plans that address specific weight management concerns.

Question 8: How can the Parkinson's Diet support overall brain health and potentially slow disease progression?

While the Parkinson's Diet isn't a cure, certain dietary choices may contribute to overall brain health and potentially influence disease progression:

- Antioxidant-Rich Foods: Fruits and vegetables rich in antioxidants may help combat oxidative stress, a factor implicated in neurodegenerative diseases.

- Omega-3 Fatty Acids: Fatty fish, flaxseeds, and walnuts, rich in omega-3 fatty acids, may have neuroprotective effects.

- Turmeric: This spice, known for its anti-inflammatory properties, has been studied for its potential benefits in neurodegenerative conditions.

- Vitamin D: Adequate vitamin D levels, obtained through sunlight exposure and/or supplements, may play a role in supporting brain health.

- B-Vitamins: Foods rich in B-vitamins, such as leafy greens and whole grains, contribute to overall cognitive function.

Question 9: Can the Parkinson's Diet be adapted for vegetarians or vegans?

Absolutely. The Parkinson's Diet can be adapted to accommodate various dietary preferences, including vegetarian and vegan lifestyles:

- Plant-Based Proteins: Individuals can obtain sufficient protein from plant-based sources such as beans, lentils, tofu, tempeh, nuts, and seeds.

- Omega-3 Sources: Vegans can explore plant-based sources of omega-3 fatty acids, such as flaxseeds, chia seeds, hemp seeds, and algae-derived supplements.

- Iron-Rich Plant Foods: Plant-based iron sources, such as legumes, dark leafy greens, and fortified cereals, can support iron intake without relying on red meat.

- Balanced Nutrient Intake: A well-planned vegetarian or vegan diet can provide the necessary nutrients for individuals with Parkinson's, and consulting with a dietitian can help ensure all nutritional needs are met.

Question 10: How can the Parkinson's Diet be integrated into daily life and sustained over the long term?

Integrating the Parkinson's Diet into daily life requires a personalized and sustainable approach:

- Gradual Changes: Making gradual changes allows for a smoother transition. Small adjustments, such as incorporating more fruits and vegetables or choosing whole grains, can cumulatively contribute to positive outcomes.

- Mindful Eating: Cultivating mindful eating practices, such as savoring each bite and paying attention to hunger and fullness cues, fosters a positive relationship with food.

- Variety and Enjoyment: Including a variety of foods and flavors makes the diet more enjoyable and nutritionally diverse. Experimenting with recipes and trying new foods adds excitement to the culinary journey.

- Social Engagement: Sharing meals with friends and family, participating in Parkinson's Diet support groups, and connecting with others who follow similar dietary approaches provide a sense of community and encouragement.

- Professional Guidance: Seeking guidance from healthcare professionals, including dietitians, ensures that the Parkinson's Diet aligns with individual health goals and nutritional needs.

Conclusion: Empowering Choices, Informed Living

The Parkinson's Diet is more than a set of dietary guidelines; it is a journey of informed choices and empowered living. Addressing common questions provides individuals with Parkinson's and their caregivers with knowledge, guidance, and a sense of agency in navigating the complex interplay between nutrition and well-being.

As research continues to unveil the intricate connections between diet and Parkinson's, staying informed and adapting dietary choices to individual needs remains paramount. By fostering a collaborative relationship with healthcare professionals, embracing personalized approaches, and maintaining a spirit of curiosity, individuals can navigate the culinary landscape with resilience, ensuring that the Parkinson's Diet becomes a source of nourishment, vitality, and informed living.

Encouragement for the Parkinson's Journey Ahead

The journey with Parkinson's Disease is undoubtedly a challenging path, marked by both physical and emotional complexities. Yet, within the intricate tapestry of this journey, there exists a profound reservoir of hope, resilience, and the potential for transformative growth. As individuals embark on this uncertain road, it becomes crucial to draw strength from within, forge connections with a supportive community, and cultivate a mindset that transcends the challenges posed by Parkinson's.

At the heart of the Parkinson's journey is the individual's resilience—a strength that can withstand the tremors, navigate the unpredictable terrain of symptoms, and confront the ever-present uncertainties. It is an acknowledgment that resilience is not the absence of adversity but the ability to persist in the face of it. Each day becomes a testament to the unyielding spirit that refuses to be defined by the limitations of a neurological condition.

Amidst the physical manifestations of Parkinson's, there exists a vibrant landscape of emotional fortitude. It is an encouragement to recognize the emotional journey as integral to the overall experience. Emotions may ebb and flow—there may be moments of frustration, sorrow, and uncertainty. However, within the depths of these emotions lies an opportunity for self-discovery, acceptance, and the cultivation of a compassionate inner dialogue.

Connection, both with oneself and with others, serves as a beacon of light along the Parkinson's journey. The beauty of shared experiences within the Parkinson's community lies in the understanding that no one walks this path alone. It is a community bonded by shared triumphs, collective wisdom, and the unwavering support that transcends the barriers of geography or circumstance. Connecting with others who share this journey can be a source of solace, inspiration, and the realization that, together, the Parkinson's community is a force that cannot be easily shaken.

Equally crucial is the cultivation of a positive mindset—a mindset that sees challenges not as insurmountable obstacles but as opportunities for growth. In the face of Parkinson's, it is an encouragement to celebrate small victories, acknowledge personal strengths, and foster an attitude that embraces life despite its inherent uncertainties. This mindset is not a denial of difficulties but a conscious choice to approach each day with resilience, gratitude, and a determination to find joy in the midst of adversity.

The Parkinson's journey is also a canvas for self-expression—an invitation to explore facets of creativity, be it through art, music, writing, or any other form of personal expression. Creativity is not bound by the physical limitations that Parkinson's may impose; rather, it is a means of transcending those limitations and discovering new avenues for self-discovery and fulfillment.

It is essential to acknowledge that seeking support, whether from healthcare professionals, caregivers, or support groups, is not a sign of vulnerability but a courageous step toward empowerment. The journey is not a solitary one, and embracing the collective wisdom and

guidance available contributes to a more informed, supported, and resilient navigation of the Parkinson's landscape.

Beyond the medical aspects, the Parkinson's journey unfolds within the broader context of life. It is an encouragement to pursue passions, engage in meaningful relationships, and find joy in the simple pleasures that life has to offer. While Parkinson's may introduce new challenges, it does not diminish the capacity for a life well-lived, filled with moments of connection, laughter, and purpose.

Moreover, it is important to approach the journey with an open heart and a spirit of adaptability. Each day may bring its own set of challenges, but within those challenges lies an opportunity for adaptation, learning, and the discovery of innovative strategies to navigate the complexities of Parkinson's.

In essence, encouragement for the Parkinson's journey ahead is a call to embrace the journey with both courage and grace. It is a recognition that, while Parkinson's may shape aspects of life, it does not define it entirely. The journey becomes an unfolding narrative—one that is rich with experiences, relationships, and the ever-present potential for personal growth.

As individuals embark on this journey, may they find solace in their own resilience, draw strength from the supportive embrace of the Parkinson's community, and approach each day with a mindset that transcends limitations. In the face of Parkinson's, encouragement becomes a powerful ally—an unwavering source of inspiration that lights the path ahead, reminding individuals that, despite the challenges, the journey is an opportunity for courage, connection, and the unwavering pursuit of a life well-lived.